THE HEALTHCARE GAMECHANGERS

12 innovators around the world reimagining healthcare

Dr. Ashwin Naik

THE HEALTHCARE GAMECHANGERS

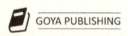
GOYA PUBLISHING

www.goyapublishing.com
Text copyright @ Dr. Ashwin Naik 2019

This book is sold subject to the condition that it shall not, by way of trade or otherwise, be lent, resold, or otherwise circulated without the copyright owner's prior written consent in any form of binding or cover other than that in which it is published and without a similar condition including this condition being imposed on the subsequent purchaser and without limiting the rights under copyright reserved above.

No part of this publication maybe reproduced, stored in or introduced into a retrieval system or transmitted in any form or by any other means without the permission of the copyright owner.

For my parents, who always believed in me enough to let me chart my own path.

And

To Priyanka and Anjalika for continuing to believe in me, while I continue my search for new paths.

ACKNOWLEDGEMENTS

This book would not have been possible without the support, encouragement and dedication of the entire team that worked with me on researching, writing, editing and polishing the stories.

My heartfelt gratitude to Farah Pathan, Sanjana Roy Choudhury, Dr. Rachita Narsaria and Rishbha Mathur who spent many hours working with me.

I would also like to thank David Aylward, Al Hammond and Sunil Wadhwani who read early drafts and were always supportive and indulgent of my requests.

Special thanks to Aditya Naik, Alden Zecha, Amit Kapoor, Anne Katherine Wales, Appaiah Mookonda, Bhargav

Thakkar, Bhargava Swamy, Harshad Bhimani, Jayesh Thakkar, Manish Sharma, Phanindra Sama, Rajesh Singh, Roma Bose, Satish Kannan, Shailesh Patel, Shanthi Mathur, Shivshankar Sanikop, Somashekhar Kerudi and Vishwas Mahajan for their support and encouragement during the publishing process.

FOREWORD

by

Stephen M. Sammut
Senior Fellow, Health Care Management
Wharton School, University of Pennsylvania

Ashwin Naik provides us with an important commentary to one of the most pressing issues of our time: the imperative that healthcare transform on a worldwide basis from its current paradigm of 'sick-care' to true healthcare. He makes his case through a litany of illustrations of innovative approaches to care in multiple countries by a dozen health entrepreneurs that dare to challenge existing models in their own countries with new constructs for addressing local needs, but with universal implications. My only regret is that the list of gamechangers is short two entrepreneurs – the author himself and his co-founder of the Vaatsalya Hospitals System, Veerendra Hiremath – who from their headquarters in Bengaluru, India have addressed the critical need of providing primary and secondary care on an affordable and accessible basis to Indians living in tier two and tier three cities. I, for one, wished that Ashwin had not been so modest as to exclude his own story. The consolation for me is the old saying: 'It takes one to know one' and applies well in this book. Ashwin knows healthcare gamechangers because he is himself the archetypal gamechanger.

This book defines game-changing in healthcare as creating connectedness among a universe of related, and unrelated, providers – sometimes new players – in fields directly and indirectly related to health. Wellness, after all, is a state of being and exists in concert with an ecosystem that provides nutrition, safe water, education, reliable energy and cultural food for the soul.

The cast of players in Ashwin's narrative represent seemingly unrelated enterprises, but this is hardly the case. The lessons from each story interweave with one another. The commentary begins, for example, with Dr. Rushika Fernandopulle of Iora Health in the United States. Iora Health's premise challenges the 'payer centric' model that has come to dominate the healthcare mindset and influence clinical decision-making. Iora assumes responsibility for a person's health, not just the outcome of a procedure or consultation. Iora's interventions occur as early as possible in primary care delivery and are able to better rationalize care and interventional strategies, thus producing healthier patients and a staff that fulfills their own vocational aspirations of delivering health.

Noora Health in India recognized early that patient care must extend from the professional and hospital settings to home and the community. When Edith Elliott founded Noora she recognized that the patient's circle of family and friends could be prepared to provide essential care during the rehabilitative period. Beyond the patient as beneficiary, this circle of new providers also raises the awareness of health practices, behavior and services in the community at large. This concept of engaging family and friends has been extended to end-of-life and palliative care by Suresh Kumar through his establishment of the Neighborhood Network for Palliative Care, also in India. The committed attention of people serving their communities in this network – even under dire circumstances – reduces complications, improves outcomes, and maximizes the benefits of care during the palliative period.

Ashwin does not pull punches when recognizing some of the inherent weaknesses in the healthcare system. He takes aims at hospitals, not on the basis of quality but on the disproportionate scope of influence that hospitals have on healthcare generally. He illustrates the alternatives conceived by several health entrepreneurs, among them Takashi Kawazoe of CarePro in Japan who sees all places where people gather as potential venues for providing care and information. This is a major shift in thinking about healthcare. While it is the case that many hospitals operate on a hub-and-spoke basis, we often ignore the fact that health and wellness depend on the fabric of daily life. Japan is perhaps the best location to experiment with this model because the attention of the population to wellness is known globally.

This notion of 'daily' and lifestyle care can also be extended from wellness to health maintenance in noncommunicable disease, in particular the growing global problem of diabetes. Morgan Guerra, the founder of Previta in Mexico focuses on helping communities build better care and support structures for people living with diabetes. In a similar way, disseminated, community-based primary care is the mission of Carlos Miguel Atencio's Medicina Familiar in Venezuela where physicians are more fully integrated into wellness.

This theme of localization must also encompass improved efficiency in care. Ashwin makes the case that the administrative infrastructure surrounding healthcare consumes significant resources in its own right, but also contributes to a 'discontinuity of care' wherein a patient may receive services from a multiplicity of unrelated providers. Even though the patient is at the center of concern of each of these providers, the exchange of information among them consumes valuable time and introduces the variables associated with miscommunication – the whisper down the lane paradox. Jos de Blok, himself a nurse, formed Buurtzorg in The Netherlands to address these inherent inefficiencies by rethinking standards of care along the lines of organizational dynamics, team structures and operations research. Moreover, the patient is brought into the picture as an orchestrator of his own care.

It should not surprise any readers that healthcare is a siloed enterprise built around competing venues for health services, as well as around today a vast array of specialties and subspecialties. The medical establishment typically rejects inputs from outsiders to the system when alternative approaches are suggested. Resisting the status quo are innovators like Joost Van Engen, the founder of Healthy Entrepreneurs in The Netherlands who has jumped borders to African countries where he established mini-pharmacies that, in addition to providing healthcare essentials, also promote preventive health through the training of local people who are integrated in their communities.

Another fresh approach to thinking about healthcare needs was in the area of breast cancer detection through routine palpation and breast examination. While self-examination is a touchstone of public health programs, few women attain the level of insight or have the sensitivity to detect lesions. Enter Frank Hoffman, the founder of Discovering Hands of Germany who realized that visually impaired people often have a hyper-developed sense of touch. Why not, he thought, train and deploy visually impaired people to serve as screeners in breast examination. This is a low-cost but high-touch intervention into a growing problem, particularly in resource-scarce settings.

Finally, a treatment of gamechangers would not be complete without addressing changing the rules of the game themselves. And this extends to bringing non-traditional resources to the setting. The story of Nalini Saligram of Arogya World in India is exemplary in this regard. Nalini had the fundamental insight that peer pressure and a sense of competition are powerful forces in all aspects of life but could be deployed as strategies in wellness, or in maintenance of health in the face of such illnesses as diabetes. Arogya World is engaged with creating corporate wellness programs driven by healthy competition, awareness, peer pressure and incentives. This is a strategy of modest cost and ultra-high impact that takes advantage of the centralization of people in the workplace. Naturally, lessons learned at work find their way into the household, particularly with nutrition.

This notion of changing the rules of the game by empowering people is put into further play by Vera Cordeiro's Saúde Criança of Brazil. Saúde Criança's program, 'The Family Action Plan' (FAP), adopts an innovative methodology: it is based on the principle that poverty is one of the important causes of disease. The plan is mobilized for intervention and follow-up care for families with sick children. It consists of a multidisciplinary team that exerts integrated actions in the areas of health, education, citizenship, housing, and income, and is built based on each family's needs. Besides overcoming the immediate difficulties inherent to the child's post-hospitalization phase, the entity's goal is to offer orientation and opportunities so that the family unit has its rights guaranteed and can enjoy a reasonable quality of life. This is a program that promotes human development through inclusion.

Finally, the rules of the prescription game are also ripe for change. Ashwin sets up this problem by observing that while the number of people being served by health systems has gone up exponentially, the service levels received have dropped dramatically. Businesses like banking and telecom innovated rapidly to meet growing demand and improve quality at the same time. Adopting the same model of serving more people in a short time in the healthcare sector has done the opposite and led to declining standards of care. Mark Swift, in creating Wellbeing Enterprises in the United Kingdom asked what's wrong with this picture and why do we continue to apply the same tired solutions to macro and micro problems expecting different outcomes? Based in the northwest of England, Mark looked at how the care of people in his community was delivered. He analyzed the healthcare profile of his local community and considered the fact that the aging population was completely reliant on the medical community for their health and wellbeing. Through a program labelled Social Prescribing, Mark's team looked at how they could develop the education of people in the community so they did not overwhelm the healthcare system with ailments that could have been treated at home, or even worse, end up with a totally preventable disease because they didn't know the effect their lifestyle was having on their body. The focus of education became lifestyle management directed at healthy practices as an alternative to the distribution of pharmaceuticals.

In summarizing the direction of his arguments and the wonderful stories in Ashwin's narrative, I have been careful not to be a spoiler for the readers. There is a richness in the telling of these stories of healthcare and wellness innovation that should not be missed by anyone who cares about the needed transformation of health systems and services. Ashwin has done us a great service in explaining how modest shifts in thinking can produce major shifts in care and improvement in health. I hope you enjoy reading these narratives as much as I did.

Stephen M. Sammut
Philadelphia, PA USA
March 16, 2019

THE HEALTHCARE SYSTEM AROUND THE WORLD IS BROKEN.

DO WE TRY TO KEEP FIXING A BROKEN SYSTEM OR EXPLORE DRAMATICALLY DIFFERENT APPROACHES?

Today, no country in the world is able to deal with its healthcare issues, from the most resource rich to the poorest. Why is it that with all the money in the world, some of the most developed countries can't fix their healthcare problem? How can countries with low resources do something dramatically different to improve health without having to spend a lot of money?

These are some of the questions I have been thinking about during my last twenty years as a healthcare entrepreneur. My most significant insight came through when I realized that the fundamental problem in fixing healthcare is that we keep trying to build solutions centered around hospitals or existing models of healthcare.

I started to think about a world where there were no hospitals. How would we then design a healthcare system? Given the miniaturization of technology and ability to connect anywhere seamlessly, it is also not farfetched to imagine that in the future, hospitals are going to disappear. Or at least in the way as we know them today. They are great for sick-care, but are in no way central to healthcare.

The next question is, if indeed the goal of the healthcare system is to keep people healthy, what is the need for a hospital?

If the goal is to treat sick people, hospitals with their complex systems, surgical tools and diagnostic machines make sense.

However, a hospital is a terrible system to keep people healthy.

They are one piece of the ecosystem, responsible for handling illnesses, when it is already late. Technology is advancing at such a rapid rate that most diagnostics and treatments will be carried out at one's home. That relegates hospitals to performing only the most complex surgeries and handling trauma related cases.

If hospitals are not going to help us be healthy, what will?

What are the new models emerging and who are the entrepreneurs behind them? Who are these emerging players that will take over the responsibility of helping us be healthy? And most importantly, what is their game plan?

The answer is fairly obvious but not simple.

In this book, we have profiled twelve such companies and entrepreneurs around the world that are building new types of healthcare organizations. We call them **The Healthcare Gamechangers**. Based on an analysis of the models developed by the Healthcare Gamechangers, four key principles seem to be emerging. These healthcare gamechangers are building their organizations around these very four principles as a key to success. And most importantly, all four principles are interlinked.

The four key principles identified are as below:

Everyone Plays: Healthcare has traditionally been driven by experts – doctors and specialists in the field. The new game, however, calls for everyone – nurses, technicians, support staff, patients themselves and their families to step up and play a substantial, if not equal, role. People who have been watching their own health and that of their loved ones as outsiders need to become truly involved in the process of prevention and recovery to take away the burden from the crumbling healthcare system.

The Healthcare Gamechanger empowers actors that are not traditionally experts, in most cases leveraging technology, like placing nurses at the center of care, empowering community members to care for each other, and train health workers to diagnose early and help in recovery.

Expands the Playground: The more that care is concentrated in hospitals, the more it will continue to be driven by old rules and notions of illness-focused care. When care goes out of hospitals and into communities, it helps expand the boundaries of what can be included as part of care. More importantly, it makes the individual increasingly accountable for their own wellbeing and not be dependent on medical experts. Breaking down the proverbial and literal walls that are cramping healthcare within clinics and hospitals will allow a two directional flow of ideas and support with the single aim of a healthier today and tomorrow.

The Healthcare Gamechanger takes a significant part of the care outside of the hospital domain i.e. to home, to the workplace, to schools, to public places like train stations and malls, and even to religious institutions.

Invites New Players: The future of health depends on new players entering this industry, challenging deep-rooted assumptions, and bringing in new thinking. Any organization focused on wellbeing has to necessarily leverage this opportunity and create an open platform for new players to contribute or participate. Playing by the old rules with the same players will not change the game. As always, the more the merrier. Bringing in other experts of say management, technology, design, and the like, is bound to bring with it never heard before solutions to traditional problems that the system is rife with today.

The Healthcare Gamechanger creates connectedness between different and oftentimes, new players, in the health ecosystem like working with organizations in agriculture, education, energy and even entertainment sectors.

Changes the Rules of the Game: The Healthcare Gamechanger organizations understand that at the core of ownership of one's wellbeing is the shift in the mindset in individuals. And enabling this is the fundamental focus of their organizations.

The Healthcare Gamechanger goes beyond illness care or preventive care of individual diseases, and focuses on a person's overall wellbeing.

In this book, we attempt to highlight innovations from all around the world and the people behind them who are already playing by the dynamic and prescient rules of the new playbook. This has important lessons for the entire medical community as how the future of healthcare industry, framing of health insurance and individual participation in handling community health should converge to contribute to shift the ill-focused healthcare to an effective health-focused system.

The Healthcare Gamechangers are:

- Dr. Rushika Fernandopulle: Iora Health, United States of America
- Jos de Blok: Buurtzorg, The Netherlands
- Suresh Kumar: Neighborhood Network for Palliative Care, India
- Edith Elliott: Noora Health, India
- Mark Swift: Wellbeing Enterprises, United Kingdom
- Dr. Vera Cordeiro: Saude Crianca, Brazil
- Takashi Kawazoe: CarePro, Japan
- Nalini Saligram: Arogya World, India

* Morgan Guerra: Previta, Mexico
* Joost Van Engen: Health Entrepreneurs, The Netherlands
* Carlos Miguel Atencio: Medicina Familiar, Venezuela
* Frank Hofmann: Discovering Hands, Germany

CONTENTS

Everyone Plays 31

Primary Care is a Team Sport. 37

Using the Rare Point of Contact to Transform Care 51

End of Life Care, Delivered with Empathy. 63

Expands the Playground 75

Care in your Neighborhood 81

Taking the Fight to the Streets 95

Retaining Doctors and the Faith of the People 105

It Takes a Community to Fix Individual Health 115

Invites New Players 131

Redesigning a Business Model to Reinvent
    an Old One 135

Solutions Present Themselves in the Most
    Unlikely Places 147

Changing the Rules of the Game 161

Connecting with Educators and Workplaces 167

Primary Healthcare is Care First, Health Second 179

Reimagining Prescriptions 193

EVERYONE PLAYS

The playing field is levelled

EVERYONE PLAYS

One of the biggest challenges in the healthcare system is that it vests disproportionate power in the hands of a few – the medical practitioners. Doctors are at the top of the knowledge hierarchy in the system and hence, wield significant power in decision-making, relegating the rest of the players to marginal roles of following orders.

A patient, during his journey through the healthcare systems across the world however, interacts with the doctors just around 10% - 25% of his time. Most of the time, the interaction is with nurses, technicians, support staff and administration. Given so much of the patient experience and wellbeing is linked to what happens in the non-doctor interaction period, it is time to question the power equation in the system.

Healthcare systems around the world are unlikely to change unless we address these issues head on. And I don't mean just more delegation to the non-doctor teams; it is truly the shift of power which is needed, the power to make decisions, the power to override decisions and ultimately, the power to set priorities for their organizations. I would wager that a truly transformative healthcare system would be run entirely by nurses, with doctors and other providers reporting to them. Of course, we need more nurse practitioners who practice primary care, more nurse administrators who run hospitals, and so on. But the key here is to build a system where decision-making or power shifts from doctors to other players in the system: a system where everyone plays.

Unless the power shift happens in a manner that it addresses these pressing concerns of power shift, awareness and preventive care, we are unlikely to see changes in the outcomes, in spite of the billions of dollars being pumped into improving healthcare each year. Unless everyone plays and towards a common goal, change is difficult.

In the following chapters you will see how Dr. Rushika Fernandopulle in the United States has built just such a system with self-organized units of nurses and customer care executives that provide primary care in their neighborhood, or how Edith Elliot is empowering patient attendants and their families to take control of their own health and be ambassadors of correct information in their communities, or how Dr. Suresh Kumar is training volunteers in the community to self-organize and care for their loved ones. Be it palliative care, preventive care or immediate care, involving everyone else apart from a doctor is the need of the hour. Each nurse, volunteer, or staff can make a difference to the life of another human being, patient or not. Every healthy person educated and made aware is one potential patient averted, perhaps one family of potential patients dodged. And though this might appear to be a small number, it is substantial when we calculate the positive ripple effect that such information can bring about.

Each of these game changers is chipping away at the old system in their own way, battling a different devil, building capacity, shifting power and ensuring everyone plays, one person at a time.

Dr. Fernandopulle and Iora Health are redefining how primary care is played out. Today, insurers tend to influence medical decision-making, which is absolutely wrong. By taking complete charge of the person's health, not just the outcome of a consultation, Iora Health is changing the outcomes right at the primary healthcare level, avoiding expensive, invasive and often unnecessary, procedures, reducing healthcare expenses and improving overall healthcare. Not just this, there is greater job satisfaction for the entire team of caregivers that attends to a patient right at the primary care level, making the person's goals for their health and life, their mission. In Dr. Fernandopulle's model of healthcare, not just the primary caregiving doctor, but nurses, behavioral coaches, psychologists, nutritionists and the person himself plays.

Edith Elliott of Noora Healthcare identified an unexpected ally in the patient's recovery process — their attendants. By training the patient's friends and family who are waiting in the hospital as the patient gets better, Edith is not just empowering the immediate caregivers with correct knowledge to reduce complications and expedite recovery, but also sending these persons, armed with accurate medical information back to the community, where usually myths and misinformation abound. In Edith's model, friends and family participate and play towards better health for the community at large.

Dr. Suresh Kumar and the Neighborhood Network of Palliative Care is breaking down institutionalized palliative care to mini local armies of self-motivated volunteers that are trained to care for those in need from their own local community. The safety net of doctors and nurses that drive the decision-making in this model in Kerala, India, is truly delivering health with care. Using the fuel that motivates volunteers each day, Dr. Kumar has channelized this caring concern to help reduce complications, improve outcomes, provide gentle but accurate palliative care. In Dr. Kumar's model, local volunteers and nurses play to give better end-of-life and palliative care to their very own community.

What Shifts when Everyone Plays

Decision making: Select few to distributed
When people organize themselves into smaller teams that can decide what's best for the people they are caring for, the care delivered is much more precise, it can address issues being missed by bureaucratic hierarchy sitting miles away, and is much faster. This can mean a world of difference as far as a person's health is concerned.

Power: At the top to the front lines
A significant amount of power is a must for every person who has a responsibility to ensure that they are doing complete justice to the job at hand. Their opinion matters.

Organization structure: Hierarchical to flat structure
A flat world might be preposterous as far the Earth is concerned, but in healthcare, it means more rapid decision-making, faster execution and individualized healthcare.

Organizing principle: Command and control to self-organizing

Having rules is great and unavoidable when dealing with masses. But if rules become suffocating enough that they choke creativity, individuality, and optimization at the cost of consistency, it's time to do away with them.

Structures: Formal employment to informal associations

The way care is delivered matters. Clean but cold environments that have all but a precisely calculated amount of care being delivered isn't the best for recovery. The term 'healing touch' was coined for a reason.

PRIMARY CARE IS A TEAM SPORT

The Story of Dr. Rushika Fernandopulle

Looking at the way things have been done in the past has limited use for the future. The medical community has developed models of health for centuries that were right for that time, dependent on the available technology and the knowledge of the health practitioners. Times have, however, changed significantly. People are suffering from different illnesses than they were just as recent as a couple of decades ago. The understanding we have as scientists and doctors of complex and obscure parts of the body are far beyond what we could have ever anticipated.

Dr. Fernandopulle is a visionary who looks at the world for the challenges he can surmount, rather than fit in line with the way things are. A Harvard Medical School alumnus, he co-founded Iora Health and is currently the CEO of this remarkable organization. Iora Health built its model on a foundation that would challenge the way things were and provide a new way of delivering a sustainable and more effective primary care system.

Iora Health's goals were pretty simple:

* To improve patient care

* To provide better quality of care from the practice

* Reduce costs

* Getting nurses, clinicians, and care managers to shift their thinking to the new paradigm of total cost of care, including the clinician's experience

At first glance, these three goals may seem at cross-purposes. It is the firmly held belief of many governments, healthcare providers and large portions of the public that to provide better care you need to pump in more money into the care system. Cutting budgets (as it would be termed in a political environment) is a healthcare no-no when it comes to political party manifestos and the way politicians court public favor when speaking to their electorate.

IORA'S HEALTH MODEL

Iora employs health coaches that manage relationships with patients on an ongoing basis, instead of looking at episodes of care and treating just the symptoms. While some interactions are remote, Iora feels it is important that the patients are met in person at least once and occasionally after that to maintain the relationship.

A particular patient had poorly controlled hypertension and type 2 diabetes. This patient developed renal damage and required dialysis several times a week to deal with this damage. In addition, the patient also suffered from anxiety and would walk out of the three to four-hour dialysis sessions, as he was unable to cope with what was going on in and around him. So, he would walk away from a scheduled session, return home to feel safe before crashing the next day and being treated with another round of dialysis as an inpatient rather than an outpatient. This happened week after week and the patient ended up being admitted thirty-seven times in one year at a cost of several hundred thousand dollars. It is simple to conclude why this was ineffective for the patient, the medical team and the client base of the practice.

That was until the patient went to Iora Primary Care, Iora Health's consumer brand. As part of their training, Iora teams looked at the patient as a whole. With the past giving quite a clear signal in this case, the health coach took the time to get to know the patient. They too felt the patient's anxiety at his home on occasions and during discussions, and so they counteracted the feeling with music. They all listened to music together, calming the patient. The health coach too listened to music with the patient while he was undergoing dialysis. With his anxiety managed, the patient no longer missed appointments and wasn't admitted to the hospital again.

In another example, an elderly patient with poor diabetes control had stopped taking her diabetes medications. She was reluctant to use insulin and had a wound on her foot. She struggled with driving and was unable to reach out to the people who could provide help. She, however, did something that changed her life. She called the office of Iora Primary Care and a physician and health coach discussed her problem. The team learned that the patient had stopped taking the medication because it would get stuck in her throat. The team talked to the pharmacist and found a drug that was smaller in size. Who would have thought that such a small change would make a tremendous amount of difference in the patient's health? But it did.

A simple conversation and understanding the patient in his entirety provided a solution that was more effective than any previous drug in addition to having no side effects and saving the healthcare system hundreds of thousands of dollars.

Patients often look for a magic bullet. They turn up at a doctor or physician and want to walk away with something physical in their hand that they can take to solve their problem. It is a natural instinct to walk in to see a doctor and want to walk out with a tangible solution. 'Take one of these pills three times a day with water after meals.' It feels like progress is being made.

But the solution more often than not is something else. The case study mentioned earlier shows that giving the patient a drug to deal with anxiety wasn't working. The physician was probably just following the norm. The normal solution for a patient presenting with symptoms of anxiety is to give them medication that will lessen the effect of the anxiety. Healthcare is currently in this rut where we look at problems in terms of prescribed solutions. Every patient is different and feels their symptoms in a different way. The solutions need to be as different and wide ranging as the patients. This takes time initially, with an associated upfront cost, but saves huge amounts of time and money in the long run because, let's face it, investing in an iPod to reduce anxiety is a far cheaper solution than patients not complying with dialysis every week or so, leading to more serious complications.

So, how does Iora Health work?

Iora Health has thrown away the rulebook that states certain symptoms require certain treatments. They have little tolerance for systems that don't look at the whole person, but focus solely on symptoms. These systems cannot be sustainable in the long term. They employ a team of health coaches that invest a certain amount of time to hear patients out and what the issues are. The idea is that Iora Health looks at the patient in a way that will keep them out of hospital and the specialist's office. The iPod example above is a great way of illustrating how this can be done.

The health coaches are selected from a wide variety of backgrounds, the primary criteria being an ability to empathize with patients and their families. 'It's one of the most innovative models out there. What they're doing is trying to start thinking outside the traditional confines of who can provide care,' says Ashish Jha, Professor of Health Policy at the Harvard School of Public Health. 'You don't need to go to medical school to be a great health coach, to connect with people and motivate them. Those skills exist much more broadly.'

In the United States of America, most employers cover employees under mandatory health insurance programs where both, the employer and the employee contribute to the cost of care. In the past, the relationship between an employer paying for healthcare and an employee looking to gain treatment has been at odds. The employee wants to try everything they can to get better. More consultations, different opinions and a chance to get better are on their mind when they walk into a hospital or meet a care provider. The doctors end up spending a lot of time trying to persuade the employer that care is needed and the patient will benefit.

The employer wants a solution, but at the lowest cost possible. They don't want their employee to go on experimental treatments or to consult several doctors for slightly varying opinions because there is a large cost involved. They want a quick solution that the doctor will find on the first visit. After all, they are paying for all of this.

Iora Health takes a lot of the 'adversarial' element out of this situation by looking at the patient as a whole and finding a solution that improves his health. This is the solution that all parties are looking for, but the way things have always been done means that it isn't the solution that is most often arrived at. Think about it in terms of pure economics. Earlier, healthcare providers would rely on patients coming back to them for treatment time and again. Iora redefines this pay per healthcare transaction model. Care teams can decide what needs to be done, and what's best for an individual, rather than picking from a set menu of what's reimbursable by insurance. As a result, the insurer pays for overall care, rather than per consultation. They charge more than a standard primary care provider to look after the patient for the insurer. But they don't look to have this patient keep coming back and undergoing the same things costing them an increasing amount of money for each visit. They look for a way to resolve the situation, or lessen the impact severely so that the patient can get back to his normal life. The future isn't one of prescribing drugs or treatment and following the path that has already been furrowed by others. It is one of managing an illness or condition so it doesn't affect the daily life of the patient as before.

Iora looks at five important things. First, it improves patient experience. Will the patient refer them to a friend or colleague? Have they re-enrolled? Second, they analyze clinical outcomes. Is the health of the patient improving? Third, they check if the total healthcare cost has gone down. Have unnecessary procedures been avoided? Fourth, is there joy in what you do? When everyone plays to their strengths in a culture of respect with a single-minded focus of patient welfare, everyone wins, including the caregivers. Last, are they staying afloat? Without this they would have to shut shop.

An immigrant from Sri Lanka, Dr. Fernandopulle was inspired by the American way of breaking rules to find new solutions. Having been in healthcare for over twenty years, he believes the current, or old, care model does not work at all. The medical industry is teeming with people that work hard for a living and have the interests of their patients at heart. There is no doubt about their dedication. But the model restricts their decisions to a simple choice: to treat or not to treat. And this decision has to happen fast. There are targets to meet, more patients to see and shareholders to appease. Each medical practice has target times, appointment times and a long queue of patients waiting to see the doctor. The pressure on time is immense. The waiting rooms of doctors and hospitals are filled with people who want their magic bullet, and more often than not, patients have busy lives and tight schedules.

The solutions that Iora Health delivers works better for everyone. The medical community gets to do what they believed they were trained for. They get to deliver healthcare that manages the problems of their patients and allows them to get on with their lives. Stories similar to the one we have come across above can be heard from doctors onboard Iora Health, about how Iora gave them a chance to do what they loved best: treat the patient as a whole and not just his symptoms.

The patients get a better standard of care. They see a future wherein their condition or illness has been taken care of or is effectively managed, often by lifestyle changes rather than prescriptions drugs with traumatic side effects. They get to feel a little bit better every day and know that they are being heard.

The people paying for the treatment, in this case insurers, get an effective solution that may feel more expensive on day one but is clearly a much more cost-effective way of managing health in the long term. People who know they are being looked after are more productive in the workplace. In a model where everyone wins, why would we ever look back to an old model that no longer delivers the results that were promised?

Iora's relationship-based care model focuses on three Ps: people, process and payment. Each patient is paired with a healthcare provider, nurse, health coach, behavioral specialist and operations team member. Each of them is deeply connected with the patient to create meaningful impact and goals that are beneficial to the patient. The process is unique in that there is a two-way exchange of ideas between all these people and the insurers to keep patient care as the sole target at all times. Using special software, incentives, special networks and marketing campaigns, Iora takes complete responsibility of the patient's entire healthcare experience, keeping the insurers happy too. Ninety percent cost reductions obtained via care at Iora Health benefit insurers/employers, and just ten percent goes to Iora.

Iora has little published research on cost savings. The company's size made it difficult to produce data with statistical significance. By end 2018, Iora was caring for 35,000 patients at 35 locations, 70% of whom are under Medicare. But researchers have compared Iora patients with similar patients in other places. Hospitalizations were down by 37% and total spending was down by 12%, compared to a control group for one of the locations. At two other locations, emergency visits were reduced by 30%.

Iora Health has raised more than $240 million since the time it was founded in 2011. The ventures investment comes from a range of technology-to-healthcare investors. As Dr. Fernandopulle puts it, their investors are investing not in us or our children, but in the future of our grandchildren. It is looking beyond today's patch-up and send back into the world, which is the biggest problem healthcare models globally are facing. Healthcare cannot be a quarter or one year's worth of investment.

Iora is also affiliated with Humana and United Healthcare Medicare Advantage plans as well as other insurances. With continued success, Dr. Fernandopulle hopes to accelerate change across the industry and open multiple similar centers across the country. Currently, it is operating in New Hampshire, Georgia, Massachusetts, Colorado, Arizona, Connecticut, and Washington.

Instead of chasing high-income patients, Iora seeks out the low- and middle-income groups and the elderly that truly need better primary care that prevents exorbitant specialist procedures and costs down the road. It focuses on doing what doctors ought to be doing in the first place: improving people's health.

The change cannot happen overnight, but the more we hear of innovative providers like Iora Health, the more likely this solution will become the norm rather than being viewed as an alternative. The effective way that patients are treated doesn't come from looking at targets and crunching more people through the system in an ever-decreasing amount of time. This just isn't the medicine that you and I know. The long-term answer is to look at lifestyle and make those simple changes early that will keep people out of high-cost care in the years to come.

The industry has a lot of work to do in this area. At the moment, it feels addicted to the way it currently works. It is an addiction that it needs to be weaned off.

Everyone plays and thus everyone benefits in the Iora Health model:

- Using client service team as the front-line workers to provide care coordination;

- Enabling care teams to take complete ownership of the health of the community;

- Using health coaches to keep the relationship-based model of healthcare at the core.

Dr. Fernandopulle feels he is giving back to society. If giving back can be so amazing, it needs to be tried by everyone.

USING THE RARE POINT OF CONTACT TO TRANSFORM CARE

The Story of Edith Elliott and Noora Health

Waiting has become an essential part of healthcare as doctors overrun appointments and people need to be ready to be seen. The appointment system leads to huge numbers of backlog every day, and the system where people turn up and wait to be seen to by a doctor can look and feel chaotic. People are there for a reason, but the wait more often than not can run into several hours if there is a sudden increase in demand for the service. As far as the hospital or healthcare facility is concerned, this is wasted time. People are sitting around doing nothing. This time is filled with communication between patients, but not communication between the healthcare team and the patients. Until the patient's name is called, there is just waiting. These are patients that are already vulnerable and need far more support than is provided to them at this stage.

In the emerging world setting, this is even more complex with limited healthcare facilities overrun with families and patients waiting for their loved ones to be attended to or to recover. Many of them travel hundreds of miles to nurse the patient and sometimes have to stay on months at a stretch at the hospital. The sickness of a family member often throws the entire family into endless rounds of hospital and doctor visits as well as sleepless nights. While doctors and other healthcare providers care about their patients, they rarely have enough time to attend to them fully, equip them with all the necessary knowledge about their condition, or how to care about it. Family members, on the other hand, care deeply but lack the requisite knowledge to take care of the patient.

Against the scenario of small budgets of healthcare provision and many patients to see, one feels there is no other way than to continue with the norm. However, as you will have already grasped till now, innovators are not the ones that accept the status quo and allow things to fester unchecked. We look at people that want to provide an alternative solution that changes things for the better.

Meet Edith Elliott. She is the founder of Noora Health and through her time practicing and researching medicine she realized during a class project that the concern and time of family members was an under-utilized asset that could potentially change the way healthcare is being delivered. Edith and her co-founders of Noora Health were working together as a team on a Stanford Design School class project titled 'Design for Extreme Affordability'. The project brought them to India where they realized that hospitals were overburdened, understaffed and had serpentine queues of patients waiting to see the doctor. Re-admission rates were extremely high too. On interviewing family members of patients, they found that they were eager to do anything to help with the patient's recovery but lacked the necessary information and were full of fear.

The team saw that the time patients spent waiting could be used far more productively and was a rare chance for the medical professionals to have contact with families of the vulnerable patients.

The question then was as to how to use this time. It was identified as present and underused, but seeing a problem doesn't solve it; it just gets highlighted. This can lead to more frustration rather than a workable solution.

The people who accompanied their loved ones to a hospital were sitting in waiting areas along with the patients. What if the idle time was converted into something productive and with long-term impact, even after they returned to their homes and villages.

NOORA'S MODEL

Noora Health uses this rare contact with financially weak patients and carers by giving them a helping hand and making a difference in their lives. These are people who have little or no education and have no access to healthcare provision, support or education in their own community, until the time they need urgent help. Noora Health delivers training to these people so they can start to understand the role they can play in preventing disease and returning their loved one to health. The waiting rooms, hospital corridors and free rooms of the care facilities are turned into makeshift classrooms and professionals from Noora address people who can have a massive impact on the lives of the patients — their own family.

These are already motivated people who want the best for their loved ones and don't want the situation to get any worse. Turning the atmosphere from one of fear while waiting to one of hope while learning is hugely positive. But the real results begin to show when people get back to their communities and share what they have learned. It creates a positive cycle of the right information being passed around from family to family. In many parts of the world, the beliefs of old rule. Families and generations pass on their learnings and knowledge. It isn't founded in the principles of modern medicine, but in centuries' old beliefs. This ranges from home remedies, to traditional medicine, to superstition all the way and sometimes to blind faith. Whatever the label, the solution is in ideas like that of Edith Elliott and Noora Health: to use the rare point of contact to pass on latest knowledge and tips to manage the health of their loved ones and neighbors which is more scientific and rigorously tested.

The initial prototype of the model was executed by a dependable nurse from their team. Initial pilots were done in the crowded and intense waiting areas of a large cardiac hospital, in an uncontrolled environment, but the difficulty was overcome by the diligence of the nurse. He delivered the materials and videos at point of service with the best of his abilities, all by himself. Once this was perfected, to scale up this approach, Noora Health converted these trainings into short videos and animations to ensure consistency in the content and the delivery. This addressed one key challenge to their model i.e., different levels of training from one-off training programs or inadequate patient-provider communication.

Overcoming this key challenge helped them build their key success factors which lies in their interactive skill-based learning imparted to patients and their families, in a consistent manner. They were able to curb the hitherto generalized and repetitive information given out by the medical workforce. They instead train and create 'nurse educators' that specialize in teaching the skills in an interesting and interactive manner.

Noora empowers these relatives with the necessary knowledge and hands-on training to take care of the patient, converting them into extended healthcare workers delivering personalized care. This takes the load off the healthcare system and enables improved recovery. Noora trains and allows the family members to practice within the safe environment of the hospital itself and helping them review their tasks on a tablet while bidding precious time at the hospital.

The training is free for government-run hospitals but provided for a fee at private hospitals. These trainings hope to bridge the gap of doctor to patient ratio which is very low at 1 doctor for 1400 patients in India, as per World Health Organization (WHO). This is a persistent problem in many other developing countries like Ghana, Namibia, and South Africa.

The aim of Noora Health is to give high-impact health skills that take little learning so people can look after their family and then their community. The advantage of this method is that people get to learn things that they clearly see can make a difference. The student becomes a go-to confidant in their community to help others manage their health. The more people out there with the skills, and the confidence to apply them, the better health standards will be as a whole.

An example of a life transformed was that of Sarathi. She was the mother of a baby boy, but the baby was at risk and his weight was low. Apart from that, Sarathi wasn't given any other information to care for her baby. In search of guidance, she and her husband attended trainings on maternal and neonatal care. After the sessions, she and her husband were confident and well equipped to support their baby. She also received materials with advice on breastfeeding and looking after her low-weight baby. It helped her to check for early signs and go for periodic check- ups.

Lives are changed because the poorest are no longer devoid of education and information about their health. Every major study conducted across the world links poverty to poor health outcomes. The access to clean water, a good diet and effective healthcare are three major factors.

Turning people from disenfranchisement is a major task, but using the fact that people are wasting precious time simply waiting in a healthcare setting goes a long way to finding a workable solution.

Figures for Noora Health prove that their system is working:

- They have trained nearly 90,000 family members in care
- They now work with 25 different hospitals
- The 30-day re-admission rate in these hospitals has reduced by 24%
- There has been a 71% reduction in post-surgical complications
- People feel less anxious about visiting a hospital because they know what is happening
- There is a 40% increase in satisfaction in patient families

These are vital outcomes and improve the lives of hundreds of thousands of people with shared knowledge. This is real impact.

Consider for a moment the impact this has on the precious resources of these hospitals. Budgets across the world are stretched to provide the best care for as many people as need it. But intervening earlier in the process, and arming people with knowledge about their health shrinks the demand on these resources. Medicine has been focused on helping those most in need of it. It is human nature to value every life equally and look at how the patient with the most urgent need can be saved. But at the same time, resources cannot be funneled away from those that are on the same path, but have arrived much earlier. If this journey remains unchecked then people will end up in the same situation at a certain point in the future. It becomes a never-ending conveyor belt of people that need urgent, and more importantly costly, care.

Noora's success shows how the forever cash-strapped healthcare system could use this informal healthcare worker system to improve patient reach, healthcare outcomes, reduce costs, as well as the burden on the doctors and nurses.

Breaking this cycle with effective and usable education lessens the chance that people will present with the same problems as their parents, grandparents or whoever else they came to the hospital with. Not only do the family members get useful advice on how to help their loved ones, they can apply much of it to their own life.

The looming type 2 diabetes epidemic that will hit the world over the next couple of decades is a prime example.

Researchers and scientists are looking at a 'cure' for type 2 diabetes. Much work and money is being injected into finding a way to reverse the condition. At the same time, people are consuming food and drink that leads them straight down the path to the condition without fail. To deal with more and more millions of people with type 2 diabetes and the related complications will blow a hole in the healthcare budgets of the world. The solution is education and a knowledge and control over eating and lifestyle habits. People need to know, and know, as early in life as possible about what type 2 diabetes feels like, the problems it causes and how to manage to keep their body away from it. The applications of Edith Elliott and Noora Health don't just exist in the poorest areas of the world; they have far-reaching benefits that could be put to use everywhere. High re-admission rates are a problem not just in the developing countries, but also in developed nations like the US which pinch the pocket of the already overburdened healthcare system. Noora is working at tailoring the teaching models for the US to help reduce the 30-day re-admission rates.

Noora's concept is simple yet extremely powerful, as it takes away the very table that separates patient/relative from the medical team that is usually on the opposite side of the table. By doing this, it makes them all a part of the same team that puts the patient's well-being and rapid recovery right at the center. Disenfranchising healthcare gives the medical workers an extended informal team while equipping the family and patient with actionable items, absorbing them into the healthcare delivery process.

This is where Edith and her organization, Noora Health are leading the fight. Going forward, their objective is to be in at least 200 hospitals by the end of 2019. This would enable them to reach more than one million families a year. They are also focusing on incorporation of experimental designs and data collection. This would further help them in developing robust methods to estimate the lives impacted and health outcomes achieved.

When everybody plays, the dynamics of the game change entirely. The sum becomes more than a mere addition of its parts.

END OF LIFE CARE, DELIVERED WITH EMPATHY

The Story of Dr. Suresh Kumar and the Neighborhood Network for Palliative Care

How we try to help people get better is changing but how we look after those who cannot be restored to complete health is also a burning subject of change.

Palliative care has, for some time now, been seen as a way of keeping people comfortable and free of pain. Of the 56 million persons that pass away each year, 44 million are in resource poor countries; 33 million of these can benefit from palliative care that encompasses physical, spiritual and psychosocial realms. As the population ages, increased longevity means that more people are living with heart disease than dying due to heart attacks. With ageing populations across the world, increase in cases of HIV/AIDS and incurable cancers, there are no two ways about it: there is a huge demand, rather need, for palliative care now more than ever before.

Many of those involved in palliative care are volunteers and this makes it far more difficult to manage. People who offer their time for free cannot be treated like a member of staff and leaned on to do more and more. Often people end up caring in palliative situations because of personal circumstances. They may have been a carer for a loved one or have seen the distress that the end of life situation can bring to people. They need this desire to be nurtured and supported, particularly if the care they deliver is to a loved one.

Looking at the patient as a whole in their last days doesn't always get the precedence it should. Quality palliative care is something that retains dignity in the face of harrowing circumstances. Today, palliative care is received as a lot to very few in the world. Of what's received, the emotional, social and psychological aspects are often ignored. The solution is to deal with the situation differently.

In the early 2000s, Dr. Suresh Kumar decided that he would look at a solution for palliative care. One of the main issues in palliative care in his home, the southern state of Kerala in India, was the cost of care. It meant that it was beyond the reach of the larger percentage of the population. People were dying at home in discomfort, surrounded by people who loved them but were unable to provide anything of quality in their care. The other main issue was the fact that palliative care wasn't covered in any great detail in medical schools in India. This is a trend, however, that can be seen across the world in medical schools.

The above two factors made it obvious to Dr. Kumar that education was the first step on this long road. Like the education systems that we looked at earlier, Dr. Kumar decided that working on this at the neighborhood level, to pass on best practices was the right way to go. The Neighborhood Network for Palliative Care (NNPC) was set up and work began in 1993.

Learning the basics of care is one thing; learning how to deliver palliative care in a different framework to what has gone before is another thing altogether. Luckily, Dr. Kumar has been able to build the network from the ground up, so every part of it works towards the same goal. Volunteers are enlisted based on the area of palliative care of their choice after a short talk on palliative care and if they are able to give at least two hours each week helping patients. The volunteers are given a sixteen-hour training course that covers different parts of palliative care and where they can fit into the team. This means that each new volunteer adds extra support to the existing Neighborhood Network.

The training isn't all in the classroom, as volunteers are given a minimum of four clinical training days with trained professionals of the home care team and asked to make home visits and examine the effective provision of palliative care. Training is offered in various aspects like basic nurse training, Train the Trainer courses, communication skills and more. It takes the empathy that a volunteer has which is then molded in the right way so they can offer care that meets the needs of a patient far better than what was being delivered. The Institute for Palliative Medicine founded in 2003 is the branch of Dr. Kumar's model that delivers the training, while the Neighborhood Network for Palliative Care puts this training into practice. It provides a connection between volunteers and professionals of the healthcare industry that can provide training and support. This is a vital connection. A volunteer help doesn't have to be amateur, so long as he/she is nurtured in the right way.

Volunteers are asked to form groups of ten-fifteen in local areas to help patients of their neighborhood. NNPC, existing local palliative care institutions, and the volunteers work together to deliver optimal care to patients. When multiple trained volunteers evaluate the situations in their neighborhood from different perspectives, they are able to discuss what they have seen with their peers, and this collective knowledge helps to build future care plans that are more practical and effective.

It switches the view of how palliative care is delivered. In much of the world, palliative care is viewed as a medical treatment. The administration of pain relief, the journey to death and the plan for that journey have all been put together by doctors. The social care element of this is tagged on at the end — as some sort of afterthought. Dr. Kumar has switched this around and has made the social aspect the most important factor in the plan. People want to help and be helped. The social aspect of the care is what gets volunteers out of bed in the morning to give help. This desire to help needs to be nurtured and honed to become the driving factor behind why people volunteer.

The medical needs are secondary. People need pain relief, but it should not be at the center of all that is going on. Palliative care primarily has social problems and thus, the society and the community need to be in charge. For people to retain dignity and have a life that is as comfortable as possible, they need to feel human. They need to feel loved.

They need to feel cared for. All of this comes from precious human time, not drugs.

Pilot testing of the program was done in Mallapuram, a low socioeconomic district of Kerala. The palliative care and long-term care coverage increased to 70% over a two-year period. Similar trends in coverage were seen in other districts like Trichur, Wynad, Palghat, Kannur and Kozhikode where the program was implemented. The networks are charged with providing support emotionally and financially, and so fundraising is an essential element of the care these volunteers provide. The Institute for Palliative Medicine has a chain of local hospitals that provide in-patient facilities while in larger neighborhoods they establish outpatient clinics to deliver as much help as possible to as many people as need it. The numbers that are now present under the banner of the Neighborhood Network for Palliative Care are pretty impressive:

- 200 neighborhood units
- 10,000 volunteers
- 60 full-time doctors
- 200 auxiliary nurses
- 2,500 patients seen per week

Care is offered to persons affected by AIDS, end stage diseases (kidney, heart, respiratory), irreversible stroke, end of life phase in old age, advanced cancers, irreversible head/spine injury, paraplegia, and chronic progressive disorders of the neuromuscular system (multiple sclerosis, Parkinson's, etc.).

Whichever way you look at it, the growth of this from a basic idea to something that is changing lives is astounding. Volunteers with no connection to palliative care are getting involved, whether a few hours here and there to contributing a vast amount of their time. The fact that they are trained and supported gets people through the door. The fact that they are appreciated and become part of the decision-making process, rather than just running errands for the healthcare staff transforms the work into something that people want to do day in and day out.

It has also changed the mindset of the medical community and the legislators. For the first time, the local government in Kerala has recognized that palliative care in the home is part of the healthcare system. Kerala is the first state in the country to have a Pain and Palliative Care Policy constituted in 2008. Unfortunately, no good deed comes without criticism and the Neighborhood Network for Palliative Care had to overcome this struggle as well. The NNPC was condemned for hiring volunteers to deliver care in an attempt to increase coverage. It was thought that this would affect quality of care. It was also feared that the expansion due to increased funding by the Government of Kerala would weaken control that the community had. The NNPC overcame the criticism by producing highly trained volunteers that met the World Health Organization definition of Alma Ata for the model of care used. They also emphasized that no medical duties were performed by the volunteers. The volunteers work closely with the community and are not obliged to any policies or goals the government might have. In fact, a large number of patients that did not qualify for traditional palliative care were now covered under the Neighborhood Network for Palliative Care. Hence, the challenges faced were turned into success factors of the program.

Getting the medical community together to support these volunteers with training and guidance keeps people out of hospital and saves money, while providing quality care that makes the patient and the family feel better. Healthcare has become disjointed over the last few decades as the specialisms have gone off on their own path without looking over their shoulder at what the rest of the industry is doing. Bringing this back together again for the final days, weeks or months of a patient's life is the way forward. It also shows the way forward to the rest of the medical community.

Looking at a system and reinventing it from scratch takes courage. Dr. Kumar decided that the system wasn't working in any way that was important to the patient. It is another classic case of the healthcare system being set up for the ease of the medical community, not the patients. But effective change brings about sustainable results that improve lives. This is what Dr. Suresh Kumar has achieved in Kerala, and is now expanding to other parts of India like Assam and Tamil Nadu and the rest of the world.

EXPANDS THE PLAYGROUND

Going out of the four walls of the hospitals

EXPANDS THE PLAYGROUND

The second challenge that is entrenched in the current healthcare system is that it is centered around hospitals, and every single process is designed is to make the hospital more efficient. However, this is the fundamental problem. We cannot define a new and radical way of building healthcare systems for the future if our point of reference is the hospital.

We have to focus our vision beyond the four walls of the hospitals, into our homes, our schools, our workplaces and our religious centers. It is time to imagine a world where hospitals don't exist and care comes to us where we are. It is time to focus on expanding the playground.

Health is not a genie that can be trapped in a bottle and made accessible to a select few. It is like scent of a flower that is experienced by anyone who crosses its path. For this, healthcare has to be taken to the very streets where the ill health is stemming from. Without nipping the problem in the bud, all doctors will be doing forever is endlessly remedying problems. There won't ever be enough doctors or hospitals or budgets. By becoming one with the people is the only way the system will survive. It is time to take every possible helping hand onboard: volunteers, nurses, families, friends and the patients themselves. It is time to take to the streets.

In this section, you will see how Takashi in Japan is taking care out of hospitals, to the busy parts of Japan – train stations, supermarkets and workplaces. You will also see how Morgan in Mexico is focused on helping communities build better primary care for diabetes and not just patients. Carlos, who is integrating community into the primary care system he is building in Venezuela, is helping both communities and doctors that feel a greater sense of contribution.

With CarePro, Takashi has overcome the challenge of waiting for the patient to come to the hospital for a diagnosis. His One-Coin diagnosis kiosks have popped-up all over malls, fitness centers, train stations, places where people spend time, often waste time. Time, the most precious commodity today, can be better utilized in making a rapid diagnosis and sharing some important information that sets the person on a path to wellbeing, much before he lands up in a hospital with complications.

Morgan's Previta Mexico has taken healthcare to the nooks and corners of Mexico. He has harnessed the power of tracking and monitoring health using technology to improve preventive, as well as immediate, care. In an already overburdened system, crushing down under the weight of the sick it cannot treat, Previta is a breath of fresh air that the government healthcare system needed. It reduces the incidence of new cases, prevents recurrence, reduces complications, reduces hospital revisits and improves outcomes for acute and chronic diseases.

A similar situation can be seen in Venezuela. Carlos decided to tackle the problem of poor healthcare and recurrences head on by going out in the turf of the patient. Using the family physician as the foundation, Fundacion Medicina Familiar is reaching out to families, not just in their localities, but in their own homes, attempting to understand the exact problems that are leading to the diseases and how they can be prevented or corrected. Instead of simply patching the person up repeatedly, they are managing to keep the patients out of the hospital entirely. And this is not just for individuals, but for entire families. For when a family is healthy and thrives, the community thrives, and as a result, the nation thrives.

What shifts when we expand the playground?

Priority: Improving efficiency in the system to wholistic engagement of community

The shifting of priority back to the patient and the community at large is probably the most important and paradigm shift needed in today's healthcare system globally. The patient needs to be put back at the center of the wheel where doctors, nurses and other support staff all work towards improving the patient's health, rather than him running from pillar to post in search of answers for wellbeing. When the focus is not the profit margin, but wellbeing and better community healthy, automatically this shift will occur.

Stakeholders: Patients and families as beneficiaries to stakeholders

Instead of looking at friends, families and the patient himself as an intrusion and obstacle towards his better health, a fresh perspective is to look at them as stakeholders. Just like any institution, all stakeholders work toward a common goal with a united vision, here, it is the patient's recovery. When combined with the forces of the medical community, the persons sitting on the opposite side of the table chip in at the responsibility of better health, dramatically different outcomes are possible, and being seen with these gamechangers. Table? If there must be one, then it must be round; a table of equals.

Dependency: Innovation on delivery rather than technology

While no one can dispute that technology has jettisoned healthcare research, leading to newer drugs and procedures, in terms of delivery of these novel therapeutic methods to the masses, there is still a long way to go. By finding innovative uses of technology, delivery of not just therapies, but also diagnostics can be improved.

Intervention: Early rather than when it's too late

Why wait till it's too late? Enabling greater accessibility to information can empower people in being their own primary healthcare provider and taking adequate steps at preventing diseases and taking timely steps. Knowledge is the single most important weapon we have to win this fight against endlessly burgeoning healthcare budgets, yet poor health and rising lifestyle disorders. If people are made aware of at least when to see the doctor, half the battle has been won.

Compliance & Behavior Change: Authority driven to peer pressure

How many times have you done something your teacher or parent said, versus what your friends said? The winner is clear. Peer pressure overpowers authority and ideals time and again especially when it comes to vital life decisions. By involving the community in its own care, we are creating an environment of healthy people, aware people. These people will influence decisions of not just their own health, but also their family's and that of their neighbors. Behavior changes don't come easy. Just like public manners, it's time public health truly goes public if we must see a different future of healthcare.

CARE IN YOUR NEIGHBORHOOD

The Story of Jos de Blok and Buurtzorg

Healthcare providers have an important decision to make when it comes to what they believe they stand for. As the world moves on with a wider range of healthcare choices from traditional and non-traditional sources both online and offline, people have a larger selection than ever before. We are in the post-information age and the fact that we can find a thousand solutions to any ailment at the click of a finger on the internet means that finding a voice as a physician or healthcare professional can be harder than ever to achieve.

Providing healthcare for people revolves around a simple choice when you look at several elements of what happens: they either deliver high quality care or look to keep costs at a minimum and make as much profit as possible. The first way isn't liked by many companies because it costs a lot of money to deliver and reduces profit levels. The second isn't what is best for patients as it reduces care standards in the chase for money. It is clear how these two parts of any healthcare business can clash and cause problems in the long run. The general erosion of standards that accompany lower costs is a worrying trend and leaves vulnerable people in a more vulnerable situation over time unless managed properly and effectively. As we look to a future with an aging population in many parts of the world, the choice is stark. We either dilute the care that we can provide with the existing budgets available, massively increase the amount of money we are spending on healthcare, or change the conventional cost vs. quality deadlock.

The more you examine the healthcare sector, the clearer it becomes that the expenditure which isn't even directly linked to the patient outcomes takes up a large amount of the budget. Receptionists, administrators, managers and others use up resources that could ideally be directed at looking after those that are sick, and in need of support or recovering from an illness or injury. But that isn't always the way how the business is structured. In addition, it takes the real caregivers, the doctors, nurses and other caregivers away from the patient, making patient-centric care an increasingly secondary motive of the organization.

In personal healthcare, otherwise known as social care, this is even more acute. Different shifts, alternative specialisms and new needs mean that some patients see a huge number of healthcare professionals on a monthly basis, some as many as fifteen different healthcare professionals that provide care at home. This produces a whole new array of problems. The patient becomes the center of the care, but not in the positive way that you might imagine these words bring. Every new healthcare professional needs to be brought up to speed with the situation and get to grips with the different care needs of their new patient. As a result, the patient often ends up directing carers to their needs, rather than a care plan or a consistency in providing and adhering to a plan. The standards of care drop while the cost inevitably increases because each new member of the healthcare team takes more time to understand the situation. The social care system is under pressure in many countries and the solution isn't just to throw more money at it.

Jos de Blok and his company in The Netherlands, Buurtzorg looked at this situation with the view that something not only had to change, but could definitely change. That is often the difference between people that spot problems and people that innovate: the ability to not just see the issue, but to study, test, research and see the solution. Buurtzorg, meaning neighborhood care, started in 2007 on a small scale and has grown into a major player in the healthcare industry that delivers results based on some simple principles. By the year 2013, the organization had 6,500 nurses working in 630 independent teams delivering care on a small-scale basis that was not only consistent for people, but had the backdrop that a large back structure wasn't needed.

By 2015, this number had gone up to 8,000 nurses with just 500 teams. Each team of nurses has a maximum of 12 members for a community of 10,000 people. This team provides care to about 50 patients at any given time of the day. With 6,500 nurses, you might expect a massive team behind the scenes of administrators, sales people, call handlers and the like but that isn't the case. The back office in 2013 consisted of thirty-five members and a team of fifteen coaches. There are now 900 teams supported by 20 trainers and 50 administrators. This is it. The nurses are able to support their own workload in terms of bureaucracy because the business model frees up their time. They don't have to rush away from a patient because they are needed to fulfil another set of appointments; they are able to spend the necessary time to assess a patient and look after their needs. This will be examined in greater detail later, but first a little about the founder and how the journey he embarked upon led to the present situation.

Jos de Blok's background can be seen to influence his present stance and the success of his company. He was a nurse and nurse manager for twenty-five years, so he possessed the knowledge of the system and its pros and cons. He loved nursing and wanted to provide standards of care that were more common when he had started his career as a nurse. It was community health nursing and was actually structured in a way similar to that of Buurtzorg today. More often than not we have to look to the past to find solutions for the present and future. Too much attention is focused on the latest technology or innovation to bring advanced results. People don't generally think that the answers to today's problems lie in yesterday's practices but the reality is somewhat different.

Later in his career, de Blok went on to become manager of a homecare organization that brought about very different challenges. He felt that a lot of time and effort was wasted on bureaucracy as management structures grew and the patient became further and further away from the reason the business operated. The care was fragmented, and schedules were planned that suited the structure of the organization or the movement of the team rather than what was vital for the patient. He became increasingly frustrated and vowed to do things differently in the future. He felt for the patients that suffered in one way or other because the standards of care were eroded by the management structure that was built to support them in the first place. Keeping a track of schedules and making sure nurses were moving quickly from one appointment to another allowed them to keep to their tight schedule but did nothing to supplement their learning, develop new ways of thinking and keep the patient well. Essentially, they just showed up, completed tasks and rushed away again. Jos de Blok knew he wanted to create an organization that took a lot of the paperwork and red tape away and delivered better outcomes for the patients over the shareholders.

He resigned from a good position and started searching for the right opportunity to put his ideas to the test. He set up his own foundation with the aim of being heavy on care and light on bureaucracy so that patients could gain a better standard of care without a huge rise in the costs.

The fact that many community healthcare companies tried to cut costs in the short term meant that their long-term costs were already on the wrong trajectory. They were lowering standards of care in the chase of higher profit margins but ended up in a low care-high cost situation because the team looking after any given patient changed regularly. This meant that the administration of the team of nurses used up more resources and became a vicious circle. This is prevalent in many community or social healthcare providers across the globe. The traditional business way of thinking in situations like this is to do one of two things (or sometimes both):

1. Increase prices for customers so the income rises to a level where expected profit is achieved.

2. Reduce overheads to a level where the profit margins are restored.

And all of this as the result of plans that were supposed to deliver better results! The solution had to be smarter with lesser red tape and bureaucracy. From a position of having worked in the industry, de Blok knew that the principle of care could be managed better if decisions of care were made by staff closest to the patient without extra levels of bureaucracy and with the patient at the heart of the decision-making process.

And so, he began.

Jos de Blok set up small, dedicated nursing teams in concentrated areas. The teams could get from place to place quickly as they didn't have to travel long distances between client visits. They knew the patients and their issues well because they visited the same ones, week in and week out. The result is lower overheads because of travel times and the removal of the 'getting up to speed' issue. The nurses were able to access the latest techniques and innovations that were relevant to their patients through the coaching team and the patients received consistent quality care from the same faces. In older patients with memory and other brain function issues, the familiarity aspect is very important and brings a better standard of care for a longer period of time.

Along with this, nurses were trusted to organize themselves. They had, after all, been through nursing programs and been trained to a high standard. Their role was to look after the patients in the best possible way and sometimes this meant looking at alternatives such as changing visit times. In the old model, this took some degree of bureaucracy and time because every change had to be put through several systems, affect several managers and could change the schedule of many nurses. In the self-managing framework, however, this wasn't the case. Decisions could be made and effected in a short period of time with minimum fuss. Patient needs were at the center of the process and the rest of the organization moved fluidly to meet this.

Nurses have a much higher degree of autonomy in Buurtzorg and are free to take decisions that are best for the patient with minimal administerial involvement. This allows nurses to have more ownership of their work and patient resulting in greater work satisfaction. Imagine this in a management-heavy organization that needs several sign-offs for any change to be enacted. Too many managers and teams are affected making even small changes which can make a huge difference to the patient, which is something to be avoided at all costs. This typically takes away the motivation with which most nurses enter the profession: to give care to a person in need. In addition, the job pays low as the aim is to reduce cost of care per hour. Thus, newer generations are reluctant to join the profession. The world just got simpler and more effective when nurses were trusted to manage themselves and their patients.

We all know that efficiency is a buzzword in management circles. But when you apply it in the simplest form, a method that actually brings real change, then it becomes more than just words. The company set up in de Blok's native Netherlands in 2007 is now growing rapidly and has been consistently winning awards for their care, three years in a row. It has managed to provide 40% worth savings to the Dutch healthcare system. This has been accomplished by reducing the hours of care to half, whilst giving an improved quality of care and increased work satisfaction to the employees.

A KPMG study from 2012 found that Buurtzorg has managed to reduce number of care hours by 50% and despite the higher cost of care per hour, it had managed to bring down the overall cost of care for patients due to the reduced number of hours needed. The quality of care per hour is much higher and the aim is not just to reduce the cost of healthcare burden on the insurance company or hospital, but to free the patient from the system eventually. This is possible because of the focus on the patient that Buurtzorg has at its heart of all care-delivery. An Ernst and Young study in 2011 reported that patients spent 20%-30% lesser as compared to other healthcare organizations. Based on this math, E&Y predicted that if all home-care organizations started using the Buurtzorg method, it would save the country two billion Euros annually!

Patients taken care of by Buurtzorg typically include those who have chronic diseases and are functionally disabled, the terminally ill, the elderly, and those recently discharged from the hospital and need some ongoing care until complete recovery ensues.

At Buurtzorg, nurses share their information and experiences with each other as well as with doctors and pharmacists through a dedicated intranet created for the organization. They learn new ways to deliver care better. The teams meet weekly to ideate and help solve problems.

Each team slowly matures into its own person, so to say, and operates as an independent unit recognized by Buurtzorg and aiming to use the collective wisdom for best possible patient care.

Buurtzorg focuses on three principles

- Highly skilled nurse teams
- Holistic home-care with teamwork
- Minimal managerial involvement

Seventy percent of the nurses that are part of Buurtzorg have the equal of a Bachelor's degree and others have a minimum of three years training. All the nurses are, without fail, highly motivated caregivers. The nurses rely on extensive collaboration and teamwork to be able to address all patient needs and make home-care as holistic as possible. Nurses reach out to the patient's families, local family physicians, general practitioners, to create simple solutions for their patients while creating awareness in the society. Some teams created articles in local newspapers while others hosted a weekly show on the radio sharing healthy habits and tips. The lean managerial teams have ensured that external factors shouldn't prevent nurses from doing their job. In spite of the 8000-nurses' strong team, there are just 2 leadership members and few administrative staff.

The eCare platform created by de Blok and a friend allows nurses to access digital records, schedule sessions and support services from other nurses. The system focuses on patient care where nurses can log into the patient's medical history and seek solutions that others might have used. This unique system has reduced bureaucratic burden by 45% on the nurses.

Another unique system developed by de Blok is the Myshopi. This shopping platform allows bundling of medical equipment, allowing competitive prices from suppliers while keeping cost of care low. Nurses can order equipment for patients from this platform. On the same lines, he is developing another system called Omaha which will allow all home-care organizations across the country to share problems and solutions, comparing their efficacy.

The Buurtzorg model of patient empowerment and self-managed patients and caregivers frees up administrative staff to focus on ways of improving care delivery and healthcare outcomes rather than spending time coordinating. It uses the patient's relatives, their informal and formal networks and relationships to aid in their care. To ensure not losing the practicality of the systems, the structures are kept simple and explained in understandable terms.

Despite the highly efficient system of Buurtzorg garnering success, it faces criticisms from its competitors arguing about higher costs and decreased quality of care. In response, the Dutch Ministry of Health, Welfare and Sport sponsored a study to compare Buurtzorg to other home health providers. The results showed a higher per-patient cost, but low overall cost of home-care services, attributed to lesser number of hours required to look after the patient. Several surveys also indicated higher employee satisfaction.

As the Dutch model of healthcare does not have a single payer system, Buurtzorg faces funding issues from insurance companies. Due to cost-containment, Buurtzorg would be disadvantaged if insurance companies base their decisions on per-hour costing rather than per-case. Another challenge is that the model grants ample leeway and autonomy to the teams. This might contradict certain government policies of employee performance monitoring. Even with such challenges in its path, Buurtzorg has been successful in spreading its model of care. The model has been taken up by Guy's and St Thomas's NHS foundation trust in different parts of England. The Buurtzorg Neighborhood Care Asia project that was set up in 2014 has now integrated community-based care in select Asian countries like China, India, Japan, North Korea, Singapore and Taiwan. The model is planning to be adopted in the US healthcare system as well.

Buurtzorg's ability to adapt to the different cultures and healthcare systems will be a test of the resilience of the model. The importance of the model may just not be associated with the growth, but also recognition of its key elements. This includes providing comprehensive care by healthcare personnel in community settings and the ability to sustain autonomous teams which eventually bring joy to work.

TAKING THE FIGHT TO THE STREETS

The Story of Takashi Kawazoe and CarePro

Time puts a lot of pressure on each one of us. There are only so many hours in a day and we all need to fit a lot of life into this finite amount of time. Work pressures are there for all to see. We all work longer hours, with longer commutes and a heavier expectation at our workplace and we continue to contribute to our company with the little extras that take time. Added to this is the pressure of maintaining a normal family life. The need to make up for sitting behind a desk all day puts pressure on us to exercise along with meal preparation, socializing, work from home, family responsibilities, and the list goes on and on and on.

There is little wonder that we leave all considerations of our wellbeing behind and ignore them until we start to feel the heat of a bad health checkup report or on how we feel physically. If it affects parts of our life then we want someone to help us feel better. If we think that we can cope with it, then we try to carry on without seeking medical help. A painkiller from the pharmacy, a heat patch from the supermarket or a few stretches and we are back to the madness. Life doesn't slow down for us, so we feel that we can't slow down for it. This is a sure shot recipe for future health problems. Doing nothing to resolve your health today just piles up problems and they erupt sooner than later.

In Japan, the pressure on time seems to be more prevalent than in many other comparable societies. The workforce is encouraged to add to the prosperity of the country and the hours worked by many are extended with social and other activities related to their company. People don't have a lot of time. The result? Four hundred billion dollars are spent per year on health care despite universal coverage. This is equal to the total tax revenue in Japan!

Takashi Kawazoe and his organization CarePro looked at this problem and thought of providing a solution. While working with diabetic patients, Takashi noticed that those that were diagnosed earlier, would have fewer complications associated with it. Most of the patients' excuses revolved around them not having the time for a health check- up, or that they never thought they were ill. Step forward the 'One Coin Checkup' method of giving a user the information that can start their journey to personal wellness. For a single 500 Yen coin (about $6) the user can get a set of readouts, where they are, including:

o   Train stations

o   Street corners

o   Department stores

These are parts of the world where healthcare is overlooked. They are parts of the world where people don't often think about their health. But there are the parts of the world where people hang out and have some time to get the connection with healthcare information that they just don't get in any other facet of their normal everyday life.

CarePro nurses are available at these places that will be able to discuss the needs of a user and answer any questions they have about the test results. People are tested for many different areas of their health, in a mere 5 to 10 minutes for as little as $5-$30, including

* Blood sugar levels

* Cholesterol levels

* Liver function

* Bone density

* Vascular age

* Lung health

This means that people can get accurate information without deviating from their routine. The wait time is only ten minutes at present for results to come back, and then there is someone to talk to about the next steps. The nature of this service is that it is quick, so people get information and advice rather than treatment, but the trigger for people to take this kind of advice or make some changes to their lifestyle is a powerful one.

There are different aspects of everyday health that many in Japan face. By focusing on this and offering a solution, CarePro has been able to make a difference to their lives. CarePro looks at people who work at a computer all day long and suffer from dry eyes or those that smoke and perform poorly in lung function tests. These are easy fixes and expand the discoverability and reputation of CarePro and the nurses that work for them.

It also offers an alternative to qualified nursing staff that want to help people directly rather than work in a hospital. Of the two million trained nurses, only one million work. Hospitals in Japan are disincentivized for hiring too many nurses. This means that the few nurses work long hours under the heavy and stringent supervision of doctors; CarePro has allowed them to use their training to help people on the path to a life of wellness. The structure of hospitals in Japan is very much along the lines of the working hours of other professionals: Tough. Because of this many are not able to attend check-ups or wellness clinics. They end up consuming healthcare when they are most in need of it, i.e. when they are very unwell.

CarePro changes the dynamics of this. Having the right information about your health is the first step on the road to doing something about it. This is a huge first step. Sheer lack of awareness that a seemingly innocent symptom might be a call for something serious brewing inside is often the reason for people not seeing a healthcare provider.

The second step to have someone to talk to, particularly quickly after the results are delivered, is vital. It strikes while the iron is hot. People are far more likely to take action at the time of discovery, rather than weeks or months later. The information and the education coming at the same time leads to a better chance of action. CarePro nurses are providing this impetus.

Even though the government provides universal health insurance in Japan, there are about forty percent of Japanese who do not receive annual health checkups. Under these social issues, the One Coin checkup is a service under which users can take their own blood sample from their finger without a doctor's presence. Due to the nature of the service, CarePro was not well received by the Japanese medical associations as self-drawn blood tests were deemed extra-legal and a threat to the existing medical institutions. This lack of understanding was fought by Kawazoe and he negotiated with the government. He made them understand that CarePro service only gives them the infrastructure to test themselves and so is not considered a medical practice. That is why they do not need doctors in this service. Their service has now been recognized by the Japanese government.

In a national committee held in 2013, Prime Minister Shinzo Abe made a remark referring to CarePro saying 'we should promote self-health checkup centers.'

After this national committee, CarePro took the initiative to develop a new policy guideline of a new classification titled 'self-checkup center', as this was a specific kind of healthcare service that did not fall under the existing regulations. Kawazoe's persistent advocacy made the government issue guidelines allowing self check-up centers.

CarePro has till now, helped more than 410,000 users in total. Fitness clubs, train stations, shopping centers and drug stores are where a CarePro counter is available.

One of such random checkups lead to the discovery of a hemoglobin A1C report being 17.6% for one of CarePro's customers. This number means uncontrolled and severe diabetes. Using the service regularly and with the guidance of the nurses, he was able to bring it down to 6%, the range for healthy people. CarePro saved his life, he says.

Convenience is at the heart of Takashi Kawazoe and his One Coin method of delivering healthcare to people when they have the time. Many people have an underlying concern about their health but don't take action and muddle through until it becomes a real problem. Takashi Kawazoe saw this and put a system in place that helps the hospitals of his country to save their precious resources in the future.

He has long been a proponent of taking the healthcare industry to the people. The four walls of the hospital are not always the place to make the biggest change. The work carried out in hospitals may save lives at the acute end of the process, but long-term care needs to be delivered in a more educational way to slow down the rate of acute admissions that is bound to increase massively if we do not make lifestyle changes or continue to deliver healthcare solutions in the same way in the future.

A sustainable solution is the one that Takashi is rolling out to the streets of Japan and India too. The costs are low and this prompts people to consume the solution that is being offered. The premise of One Coin is a great one, and married to high-quality service, it is a winning offer.

CarePro aims to not just prevent lifestyle-related diseases but also reduce medical expenses.

The Impact

In India, 3 out of 100 made an appointment with a doctor after seeing their results.

Sixteen percent people said they planned to come back again later.

Getting people increasingly confident about their health and being able to manage it effectively is the end goal for all those that work in supporting others. Solutions like CarePro take the power out of the hands of the hospital and puts it in the hands of ordinary people. In the past, we would have had the skills and knowledge to look after ourselves. This is now eroded and we rely on the skills of others to help out. But even then, we seek out this help when it is too late. We end up taking drugs for completely preventable diseases rather than having the knowledge to take the steps that would have stopped them from happening in the very first place. The future looks very different to the past. Getting information about our health is the first step on the road to recovery. CarePro's nurses take you two steps of the way.

In Takashi's innovation, everyone plays improving not just access to healthcare but reducing unemployment in the healthcare industry while addressing pressing healthcare needs of the nation.

RETAINING DOCTORS AND THE FAITH OF THE PEOPLE

The Story of Carlos Miguel Atencio and Medicina Familiar

Access to healthcare is a global issue but the solutions are largely local and contextual. Every part of the world faces its own healthcare problems. In some countries, there is immense pressure on decreasing costs while in others systems are falling apart because of a paucity of general and trained staff coupled with greater need. Particularly in countries that have low budgets and a heavy level of interference from the government, medical professionals tend to seek the first opportunity to escape from that level of burden or interference. The work becomes futile in their eyes and the future doesn't look any different.

In medical circles, helping people is often referred to as a calling rather than a profession, but there are limits as to how much can be done on a small budget. Seeing the same patients time and time again with the same issues doesn't do anything for the morale of the workforce. They feel like firefighters and don't get to make the interventions that change behaviors and deliver people to a healthier way of life.

In Venezuela, the above two issues happen all too often. Healthcare professionals train to a very high standard and are then let down by poor resources to be able to help people. From this outcome, they become disillusioned and look elsewhere to work. Like English, knowing Spanish is a passport to work in large parts of the world. Venezuela sees six of every ten doctors leave their healthcare system after being trained to other better-funded Spanish speaking countries. Seats in medical schools are going vacant while the citizens struggle to get better healthcare. The doctors that do stay back opt for specialties that enable private practices with higher incomes, like plastic surgery or ophthalmology. The massive amount of money spent on training doctors and nurses is eventually a waste that could be put into patient care, effective patient care at that. This catch 22 situation means that more money is ploughed into training, leaving less for patients, so more doctors and nurses leave, and we continue on the same slippery path.

Carlos saw this problem every day in his work as a doctor in Venezuela. Venezuela spends about USD 90 per person each year on healthcare. Of this, roughly over a half (USD 50) is government funded. This is far from the USD 1860 that developed countries spend on healthcare and also lower than the USD 105 that other Latin American countries budget for their citizens. Reduced budgets meant that a lot of healthcare facilities were centralized and people had to travel a long way to go to the hospital or visit a clinic.

People didn't participate in their own care until they were so ill, they needed hospital treatment. From there, they would return home and go back to being disengaged with their health until another major problem cropped up. It wasn't healthcare as we know it; this was walking into the same problem day in, day out. Costs were going up because the severity of the patients was higher and there was no future other than one where people got sicker and doctors worked longer hours for the same pay. A recipe for utter disaster.

About 25% of the population of Venezuela needs some medical attention each month; of this a meagre 1% needs intensive or specialist medical intervention that requires cutting-edge technology, a surgery or hospitalization. Coupled with the dearth of primary healthcare providers, this only means that a patient relies immensely on specialists instead of integrated and preventive care. This scales up the cost of healthcare due to unnecessary tests, making healthcare increasingly fragmented and burdening the already overburdened healthcare system.

Carlos didn't want a future like this. He saw a different way of dealing with the problem. And he acted. He decided that the centralization of care in a hospital was at the root of the problem. If they were detached from the community, then it was little wonder that the community was detached from them. The people they purported to help were the very people that they had abandoned in many ways. Healthcare in Venezuela became associated with sickness instead of being associated with wellness.

As already discussed, this is something that needs to be worked into the attitude of people more than the care that they are given. Education is a wonderful thing and delivering it in the heart of the community changes attitudes far more quickly than doing it any other way. And so Fundacion Medicina Familiar (FMF) was founded by several physicians, business and community leaders, with the aim to prevent people from getting sick in the first place. A pretty simple and noble aim.

The FMF model is reviving a dying 'specialty' i.e. family medicine/general practitioner approach with preventive and primary care that is based on proximity to the patients and integrated medical knowledge. Since it is a community-based model, a doctor also visits the patient's home, which helps both to maintain a record of healthy habits and progress of healing process. The guidance given to patients is either at very low prices or free depending on the financial status.

Firstly, they got in closer proximity to their patients by taking over clinics in the locality. Rather than expecting patients to come to them, they went out and met people on their own turf. The hospital system of silos where different specialists knew different things was great when dealing with acute problems in specific areas of medicine, but didn't look at it holistically. By definition, a specialist has detailed knowledge about one subject in particular, but little knowledge about other things. This would mean patients being passed around different hospital departments for different solutions.

In contrast, Fundacion Medicina Familiar used general practitioners (GP)/family physicians (FP) to help people with the wide-ranging issues they faced. Simply put, if a specialist referral is required, it can happen, but the whole person was considered by the GP/FP. They started to educate people in what they could do to make their life better. Patients learnt about the changes they could make in their life rather than wait until they were in acute need of medical attention. Not only did the GPs help the people in the local community, they also took a great deal of pressure off the hospital because:

- People didn't turn up at the hospital with lesser ailments because they had no idea how to deal with them

- People were better able to manage their health to stay away of hospital completely

And these are meaningful solutions that changed the life of the people in the poorer parts of the cities of Venezuela. It isn't necessarily about getting a larger budget to make a difference in health. It is more often than not about using that budget in the right areas to get people better without the need for acute care.

The Impact

The foundation has been able to provide free medical care to a population of more than 6,000 people of whom 80% still live in poverty. They have impacted over 2,000 people with its community activities by educational and health promotional actions.

Nearly 5,00,000 patients have come through FMF health centers in the last five years, and 11 universities have begun offering courses in family medicine.

Fundacion Medicina Familiar now has a team of seventy medical professionals looking after patients in their own community from four health centers in the country. This has allowed doctors and nurses to feel more connected to their patients as they can see a marked improvement in health. And guess what? This has meant that Venezuela has been able to retain their healthcare professionals because they realize they are making a difference, whereas earlier the futile nature of 'patch them up and send them home' was forcing Venezuelans to look elsewhere for fulfilling employment opportunities. The future of helping their fellow citizens to wellness has prompted a much higher retention rate in the Fundacion Medicina Familiar team than was seen before.

Getting into the heart of a community is the perfect place to make a change. People want to look after themselves, which is a fundamental aspect of human nature, but they too often don't know how. Initiatives like Fundacion Medicina Familiar put the power back in the hands of the people. As they understand what they can do to enact change in their own life, people assume responsibility. This can be a little frightening for doctors that have seen their control uninterrupted but it enables the medical community to focus on the cases where people just can't help themselves. Unfortunately, there will always be accidents and sudden illnesses that fall through the care of the GPs, but the beauty of this system is there will be far fewer of these cases.

The FMF team consists of both administrative staff and medical professionals led by an administrative manager, medical manager, program director, and human resources director, all based in Maracaibo, in northwestern Venezuela. Spread among the four centers are nearly fifty doctors and twenty nurses and a team of volunteers, mostly from the UNIMEFA Association that helps with administrative tasks and general health promotion within the community.

The FMF model is based on four pillars, each intentionally addressing a different barrier in the current health system.

The first pillar is continuity and integration. The health center is located in the community it serves. The center takes regular appointments for outpatient care but also has an emergency service, and is always available to attend to patients. Second, the same health team, comprising a doctor and a nurse, always attends to the same individual or family, both for routine checkups and for graver problems. The idea here is that the team is familiar with the patient and his or her health history and helps in building trust.

The second pillar is productivity and sustainability. FMF staff is paid according to the number of cases they see. Patients pay a fee, but the cost is 50% - 70% less than what the procedures would cost in private health centers. A small percentage of this fee goes into a fund to subsidize community patients that are unable to pay for their care. This not only reduces the cost of care to the patient directly, but also keeps responsibility on the shoulders of the caregivers.

The third pillar: Carlos has developed a training and evaluation system to ensure consistent quality in FMF care. All of the medical professionals at FMF are trained in Primary Health Care. Doctors receive a post-doctorate in family medicine from the University of Zulia, which also offers continuing education in person and through distance learning. Carlos has designed an evaluation system for each aspect of the center. FMF uses indicators measured on a monthly basis such as productivity, financial health, and satisfaction. User experience is critical, so surveys question all stakeholders, patients, staff, and the client companies.

The final pillar is community participation. FMF is governed and monitored in part by an association of other community organizations, called the Unidad de Medicina Familiar or more popularly known as UNIMEFA. Other groups, such as Alcoholics Anonymous and the secretary of Culture, also organize health-related activities in conjunction with FMF. The patients themselves monitor the quality of the care through their hand in governance and evaluations, but also through these trainings and seminars on health topics, to learn to take care of themselves and be responsible for their own wellness.

Carlos has allied with several public and private sectors to increase its success. Several foundations also support the cause. The Medical Association of Rescarven has adopted the Family Medicine model and trained doctors across Venezuela. With help from the government at the regional and national level, Carlos has successfully expanded the model and tried to transform the face of health centers.

Today, FMF general practitioners can treat 85% of health problems they encounter leaving only 15% to be tackled by specialists or larger centers. Carlos estimates that focusing on preventive care, early detection and personalized primary care, the current cost of private healthcare can be brought done by a whopping 80%.

Healthcare has become about sickness far too much in society as a whole. We go to seek help at the wrong time. If we prevented, rather than cured, then a lot of the strain would be taken off the healthcare systems to develop in the right way. But this takes education. And education entails looking at things differently.

IT TAKES A COMMUNITY TO FIX INDIVIDUAL HEALTH

The Story of Morgan Guerra and Previta Mexico

The idea that we must treat diseases such as type 2 diabetes by focusing on early detection and diagnosis is the predominant model of care around the world. The focus of the medical community is to ensure early and rapid methods to achieve the following two objectives:

1. **The initial discovery of a patient with type 2 diabetes:** This involves the support needed to manage the disease.

2. The complications associated with type 2 diabetes: This can involve more radical interventions than advice, such as surgery.

The medical community handles this relatively well. They are able to identify the condition, hand out basic disease management advice as well as perform interventions for those that have developed other health problems as a result of their diabetes. But this, for me, is a very narrow view of how healthcare should be delivered.

Some information leaks out to the people around the patient when the information in number 1 above is delivered and when the procedures in number 2 happen. To break this down, the patient receives information about how to manage type 2 diabetes, and possibly how they may have developed the condition. Their friends and family will also learn a little about the disease at the same time. When the patient with diabetes goes through a major intervention such as surgery, their friends and family experience the shock of seeing a loved one at risk. Initially, you would think that these two factors would have an effect in lowering the occurrence of type 2 diabetes in the patient's family. But the fact is that people with type 2 diabetes in the family are more susceptible to contract the disease. It is the environment and associated habits that people live in which determines their likelihood of developing the disease.

As a medical community, we need to stop and think about how effective the treatment we deliver is actually going to be and how to better it. If we advise someone to manage their own condition, then why isn't this percolating effectively to the people closest to the patient? Why are we looking through a kaleidoscope at the patient alone, and not at the whole family or community at large that can benefit far more from the kind of medical attention that stops diseases such as type 2 diabetes from happening, than the current model? The words 'something has to change' have been used many times in this book. I hope that by now the reader will agree that there are better models out there if we look at what some innovators are delivering, often in difficult circumstances and with negligible resources.

The effect of type 2 diabetes on the life of a person who is newly diagnosed with the condition changes beyond all recognition, especially if not managed in a proper manner. But the disconnect between the patient and the doctor is such that they are only placed in the same room when it is usually too late. This is the model of illness that we are trying to move away from. This is the model that will see a huge pressure on its services in the future unless a radical change takes place now. And that is where the issue often lies. The model of future healthcare looks radically different when compared to the way healthcare is currently delivered across the globe. We must stop waiting until it is too late.

Morgan Guerra is an innovator who is working to change this model. He works in his native country of Mexico delivering healthcare to entire communities at once rather than focusing on those that are unwell enough to arrive at the door of the hospital. Morgan has taken the fight against chronic diseases such as type 2 diabetes, high blood pressure and obesity, to the streets. He has moved the focus away from the hospital and illness to the health status of the community.

As mentioned earlier, this approach feels radical in comparison to the current system, but looking at it with a fresh pair of eyes, this is the way toward a healthier lifestyle. Morgan has worked in many different aspects of the healthcare profession and has developed his ideas of the way it should be delivered. He has seen members of his family fall prey to chronic disease and looked on in utter shock at the resources and attention that managing a disease got, when the more effective way of spending money was to go out into the community and work on prevention. It is a better way to spend the healthcare budget as:

- It is far more effective at preventing disease
- It costs less money in the long run to keep people healthy than it does to mend them
- It allows people the confidence and skills to manage their own health; a greater buy-in gives better results

- It is more engaging and fun than the current model
- It reduces the risk of the disease in the community

All in all, there is a move towards making the lives of people better with the kind of model Guerra successfully uses with people in his community. The lack of engagement with the medical community from the average person is alarming. There is so much they can learn. But we have come to associate healthcare with those in the greatest need. When we are asked to think of the kind of people that use a hospital and the services it offers, we will think about those involved in an accident, those that require a surgery and those that have developed chronic disease. What if we could change that perception? What if we could get people to think of doctors as those that managed people so that they would stay fit and healthy? What if we could get people to engage before they became sick, to prevent becoming sick? The new model would change the life of millions of people across the world. For a start, it would stop the masses from developing type 2 diabetes.

According to the World Health Organization (WHO), the number of persons with diabetes has risen from 108 million to 122 million between 1980 and 2014. In 2016, nearly 1.6 million deaths occurred across the globe as a direct result of diabetes. Its prevalence is increasing sharply in low- and middle- income countries like

Mexico. Over 12 million adults in Mexico battle with diabetes each day and this number is expected to rise to 16 million by 2030.

Back in 2017 itself, the government of Mexico declared diabetes a national emergency, which is huge for any country. Amongst the 35 countries in the Organization for Economic Co-operation and Development's (OECD), Mexico has the most diabetes-related hospitalizations as reported in 2017. In spite of the National Strategy for the Prevention and Control of Overweight, Obesity and Diabetes that is in effect since 2013, Mexico is fighting the deadly epidemic on three fronts: public healthcare, medical aid, and regulatory policies. It spends big money on treating those with type 2 diabetes. The financial burden of type 2 diabetes was about $860 million pesos in 2013, equaling the 2.25% Gross Domestic Product (GDP) of that very year; a sum greater than the real growth of Mexico, 2.1%, at 2014 end. This money has to be raised from somewhere and taxpayers, the people themselves, are the prime source. At the same time two other factors are at play:

1. There will be people who fall through the cracks. Those in the poorer communities always seem to be at the top of this list.

2. There are more people all the time contracting diseases that adds to the pressure on the system.

A large number of Mexicans are detected to have diabetes at a much younger age as compared to other OECD countries. Nearly 3.25% of cases are detected between ages 20 and 39 as compared to an average of 1.7% in other OECD nations, according to a recent review. This means that the new generation is not learning enough from the suffering of their elders. Continually monitoring whole communities to see if they are becoming more susceptible to chronic disease looks an almost impossible task.

The current healthcare model has neither the desire nor the budget to be able to add this task to the thousands it already carries out. So, more people will be coming down the line for care and more vulnerable people will be ignored and endure a painful existence without the support they need. This isn't a sustainable way to look at the health problems we face as a society. Unless an intervention is made much earlier in the process of wellness to sickness to treatment, we will end up with a conveyor belt of the sick hitting hospitals in ever increasing numbers for the future. The decision then has to be whether to increase healthcare spending exponentially to cope with this, or to cut some people out of the system altogether, that is to deliberately let people fall through the cracks. Of course, this will fall on the poorer sections of society. This cannot be the future we have planned for the planet.

Morgan Guerra views the future differently. He is looking at the interventions needed and making them happen in his community in Mexico. And technology plays a major part in realizing this. Guerra is taking the healthcare to the people rather than waiting for them to turn up at the hospital.

Previta constantly remote monitors patients and gathers data for preventive health. It has a three-pronged approach to the ailing healthcare system in Mexico:

- It treats the entire community as a whole using high end technology and tracks patients with specialized software
- It uses doctors as health coaches
- It has a multidisciplinary team of specialists

Guerra uses mobile units and cellular phone technology to have teams on the streets which allows people to submit data remotely to a centralized office. This provides his team all the information they need to remotely deliver effective healthcare that changes the lives of entire communities and will take the pressure away from acute care in burgeoning hospitals in the future. Previta has an e-Health Tracker platform that provides service to the doctor and the patient. The entire medical data of the patient gets stored in the application, which in turn gives the doctor an opportunity to access it remotely. It effectively uses remote tools like mobile units and telemedicine technology to enable doctors to give consultations with ease. These systems have been built keeping in mind the high density of patients and at-risk persons of chronic diseases in semi-urban and urban areas. Around 500 doctors and 150 offices have implemented it.

The Impact

- Seen over 200,000 patients in the first 9 years itself
- Reduced over 15% total healthcare costs of the populations it serves

It is a model that looks at helping the well and the sick. It takes a whole community and monitors how they are acting in health terms. Looking closely at the lives of the people who are close to a patient who presents with a chronic disease, they are in the same environment, facing the same conditions; they often lead a very similar lifestyle. Their chances of developing the same disease are high because they are exposed to the same conditions as the patient who has already developed the condition. In fact, the whole community is. So why not look at the community as a whole? Previta does exactly this.

Previta looks at how it can help people to understand their health through a team of doctors it calls 'health coaches'.

These health coaches are ready to answer questions of patients and their family at any time, remotely, using telemedicine. They are armed with the information from remote, constant monitoring and can look at different parts of the community to promote healthy living and give advice when needed. This helps doctors as well, as patients have greater control over their health (and illness) and minimize complications. These health coaches are responsible for patient training and are the primary point of contact between the patient and Previta.

There is a multidisciplinary team of specialists too onboard Previta comprising a nutritionist, cardiologist, general physician, endocrinologist, psychologist and ophthalmologist. While such specialists are irreplaceable in any effective healthcare team, it is important to differentiate the roles of a specialist and a general physician. High rates of doctor unemployment are seen in Mexico due to saturation of the market with specialists and not enough general physicians who end up working in corner pharmacy stores for lack of respect in the community. Previta's digitization of healthcare is enabling these doctors to use their training and bringing in a new breed of doctors that are familiar with e-medicine.

Engaging the community in their own healthcare is a paradigm shift in the way hospitals deliver care at the moment. Previta helps people who are well or at-risk to look at their health differently. Their mobile units have trained personnel who do a basic physical examination, patient education about their healthcare concerns, identify goals for treatment and draw up follow-up plans and most importantly, identify compliance barriers, promote including the family in the treatment, and create actionable plans for patients customized to their lifestyles. They spend time with people, while they are healthy talking about their goals, their values and their fears. They plan educational activities for healthy members to prevent illness. These plans are available online so that the member of the community can access it at all times. The plan helps people to focus on what is important and to be able to manage their own health. They get access to information that provides them a framework to stay healthy and away from chronic diseases that might otherwise have been in store for them. People who understand and have the confidence to look after themselves are far less likely to end up in hospital with a major illness. A vast majority wants to be able to look after themselves, with a little nudging from their medical practitioner, rather than close their eyes and hope that someone can patch them back together again if there is a problem. Previta gives people these skills and gently prompts their action through SMS reminders, online monitoring and the support structures that don't exist anywhere else.

Guerra has expanded the playground to the entire community and torn down the metaphorical walls of hospitals that cloister healthcare. He has taken the doctors to the ill and the well to prevent sickness. This prevention is not just helping reduce the burden of sickness in the society but also the cost of healthcare the society itself has to bear, and the burden that the few doctors have to bear. It is improving overall wellness quotient, reducing morbidity and death rates, reducing the risk in at-risk persons, preventing complications and slowing down the course of disease in those who are already diagnosed with a chronic disease like diabetes or high blood pressure.

This is the difference that makes Previta effective. People are supported. Turn up at a hospital with a detached retina and a highly-skilled surgeon will reattach it for you. The wonders of modern science are there for all to see. But what if people were given advice on how to manage the health of their eyes to reduce the chances of this happening? The world looks different all of a sudden. Previta provides this service to a million people a year. It has also reduced the healthcare costs for the people it serves by around fifteen percent so far. Prevention is better than cure because it is also cheaper and improves the overall quality of life.

Stopping a disease from happening is a cheaper way than waiting for it to happen and dealing with the consequences.

INVITES NEW PLAYERS

Opening the doors to play

INVITES NEW PLAYERS

The next challenge in healthcare is the siloed approach to care, with no interaction or collaboration with outsiders. The technical aspects of medical care are so complex that the industry is hiding behind its own four walls. But technology is changing rapidly and is enabling the system to open to people outside the industry – engineers, physicists and philosophers – to come in and shake things up. And not just to bring their technical expertise to build the next gadget or improve the diagnosis, but also to fundamentally challenge deep-rooted practices of the way things are done. I am convinced that the future of healthcare delivery rests on how easy we can make it for others to participate and contribute, and not just be alarmed by the inefficiency and lack of progress from the sidelines.

The central issue here is not lack of interest from outsiders but our own mentality of building walls to keep everyone else out. One of the most common refrains you will hear in the medical community is, healthcare is different, it's not like other industries. Well, every industry used to think this way till someone just decided to do something about it. And we know from history that most innovations which shook the world came from outsiders, in some cases non-experts. The Wright brothers and the airplanes are an excellent example, where they competed with the world's leading mathematicians and thinkers to build a better system. They were not constrained or shackled by preconceived ideas. They were naive enough to not know what is not possible.

Maybe healthcare needs such persons too, with an open mind and a can-do attitude to renovate the system. Maybe it's time to invite new players inside the four walls of the hospitals and the minds of people in the healthcare industry.

In previous sections we have discussed how breaking the rules, writing new ones, expanding the reach and making everyone participate is changing the game. By welcoming a fresh perspective at running the show, they are showing how healthcare can be done differently. Be it Joost van Engen in The Netherlands who is working with communities in

Africa or Dr. Frank Hofmann who is giving a harnessing to the power of the visually challenged to improve breast cancer detection, they are bringing in new people aboard the ship that seems to be sailing away.

Healthy Entrepreneurs is empowering locals from various African countries to start mini pharmacies in their communities where they don't just sell important healthcare essentials, they are trained to be ambassadors of preventive health in their locality. Providing them a livelihood, self-respect, and basic medical knowledge is reducing morbidities in the communities where these mini pharmacies exist. And who are these locals who are chosen? They are everyday folks with no medical background whatsoever, just the will do something productive, learn and earn.

Dr. Frank Hofmann harnessed the superb sense of touch that those with partial or total blindness have to detect breast cancers. Discovering Hands has given not just many women with breast cancer a new lease on life by early detection, but also enabled a life of dignity, growth and respect for the visually challenged.

What shifts when we invite new players?
Frameworks: Dogmatic to try something new

When we break the old mould and set out on a new journey, we are bound to find new opportunities that might give us the answers we are looking for. Shedding dogma can change healthcare outcomes dramatically as we can see clearly in the game-changing routes taken by Dr. Hofmann and Joost van Engen. Making the impossible possible is a challenge that can be fulfilled only by those that are ready to go to any limits and are driven by a passion to truly see a different future than one we imagine today.

Scope: Look in familiar spaces to explore the unknown

Have you ever searched in the same cabinet for something and not found it, but your mom has? Sometimes we don't find what we are looking for despite searching for it in a well-known space, but a person with zero prior exposure may find a hidden gem right there, amidst all the mess. This is what healthcare is looking for today. These innovators are like the mom that can find something precious amidst all the clutter in your cupboard just when you need it the most.

REDESIGNING A BUSINESS MODEL TO REINVENT AN OLD ONE

The Story of Joost van Engen and Healthy Entrepreneurs

The world over, money is at the center of much of the healthcare provision. Making people better when they are sick is big money. Even in countries where healthcare is free at the point of delivery, such as the United Kingdom, there is a heavy price to pay. In a country of approximately 65 million people, the National Health Service (NHS) budget sits at around $130 billion per annum. Multiply this by the number of countries in the world and you can start to see that the annual global spend on healthcare is a huge sum. And everyone wants their cut. In the modern-day business model, every company looks to make as much money as possible with as little expenditure. This may look like solid economic sense, but you have to ask the question whether this crosses over as a viable model for a healthcare business. The jury is out on this. But the choice doesn't have to be between a highly geared profit-making machine or not-for-profit; there can be a middle ground.

One of the ways that healthcare has closed its eyes to progress over the last twenty years or so is, to new ideas. They innovate in terms of looking for new treatments of drugs, but not in the way that these are delivered. A hospital is still the center of excellence and information in just about every part of the world. It hoards the best doctors, the best nurses and the best practices. It feels like it should be able to cure all ills, so invites people to visit if they are unwell. The center of excellence looks after its own. If you go for treatment you will be offered the latest techniques, the most sophisticated treatments and the newest prescription drugs on the market. Then you are sent on your way. We have seen so many times in this book that this isn't the way forward.

But we can learn from business. If you look at the business community, then it feels dominated by the big players.

Look at the financial news and in the markets and all talk is about the top one hundred companies, the big takeovers, the billion-dollar deals. But once you scratch the surface then you will find that the economy is made up of companies that are many different shapes and sizes. The small businesses may only employ a few people at a time, but together they contribute a lot to the economy. There are medium-sized firms that grow steadily over a number of years to provide good service to their customers. They are happy making a good living while serving others, and don't have the aspirations to make billions of dollars in profit year after year. The people of the world, the real people, look to this vision of the future with dread. They will become hostage to either the healthcare community or the health insurance community. This isn't the way ahead for regular people.

Small- and medium-sized companies need to emerge that will challenge the big players and break the monopoly of the hospital. The hospital is a great place to go if you are very ill indeed. But what about those that are quite well, but want to prevent sickness? Where is the provision for them? What about those who are living in the poorest parts of the world? They have been left behind by expensive healthcare or the rising cost of insuring your health. What about those who live in remote parts of Africa or Asia or South

America and live far away from a hospital to travel on a regular basis? Who looks after them?

The African region houses 11% world population but 60% persons of people diagnosed with HIV/AIDS live here, which remains the leading cause of death this region. Over 90% cases of global cases of malaria occur in Africa each year. Of the 20 countries that witness the greatest number of maternal deaths, 19 are from Africa. The highest newborn death rates across the world are in African countries. The burden of infectious as well lifestyle diseases on the African health systems remains high.

Joost van Engen saw this problem far too often. He saw many of the problems that we have been outlining in this book:

* People on low incomes without access to healthcare

* People who lead unhealthy lifestyles but have never been given the information to change this lifestyle

* People who don't manage their bodies, but rely on emergency care when they have an acute problem

There is little access for the poorest in society for even the most basic of healthcare education messages around alcohol, nicotine and diet. This means that people are already walking headlong into a situation they don't know anything about. The result is that totally preventable diseases are ravaging parts of the world. People are turning up for help at the wrong time in the process. If they knew the dangers of excessive sugar, for example, then they would have been able to change their diet and lifestyle to reduce their chances of developing type 2 diabetes.

Disconnect between the person and their health seems to be at the highest level. People are not educated about how to look after themselves, their children, their families and are put in danger every day of their lives because of this. We move away from the 'Western' diseases caused by excess, and look at how other people on this planet have to cope. They don't understand:

* Basic hygiene that prevents them from getting infections

* Contraception that will stop them bringing more children into unsafe conditions

* Abortion practices that leave the mother in a very vulnerable position

* Safe sex that will stop the spread of diseases such as HIV

Healthy Entrepreneurs (HE) focuses on the need of emergence of small- and medium-sized companies. Joost van Engen looks forward to have different means of delivery of drugs rather than just innovate in terms of looking for new treatments of drugs.

What does Healthy Entrepreneurs do? Healthy Entrepreneurs themselves manage the end-to-end distribution chain. This ensures that quality of the supply as well the products remain low cost as opposed to where the suppliers keeping high commission. Joost aspires to set up healthcare companies that are happy making a good living while serving others. His vision is to provide and serve those that are medically fit but want to prevent future sickness. And to provide healthcare to those that are living in the poorest parts of the world as they have been left behind by expensive healthcare or the rising cost of insurance.

Attitudes are sometimes difficult to change, but they are impossible to change without any information getting out there to the people that matter. There is a kind of lawlessness when countries that are inherently poor have people that need access to healthcare. The hospitals suffer from low levels of investment, leading to unhygienic conditions, a lot of pressure on services and no education delivered. They are centralized, so people in the remote parts of the country miss out. The World Health Organization (WHO) estimates that between 10%-30% of prescription drugs in the developing world are counterfeit. The system lacks the sophistication in detecting the counterfeiters, the smugglers or the runners as there would be in a country with a larger budget.

The model that doesn't work in the developed world is totally dysfunctional in the developing world. It leaves people out of the loop in many places. It fails the people of these poor countries in many ways.

Joost Van Engen decided there needed to be a change, and through his organization he looked at the supply chain of healthcare to the poorer people of countries such as:

o   Rwanda

o   Burundi

o   Uganda

o   Haiti

People in the supply chain want to make money, which is the nature of business. But Joost van Engen was looking towards the small- and medium-sized players, just like we considered in business, to become stakeholders. This way the people at the end of the supply chain got access to education, medicine and support while all the others made money, but not at ridiculous profit levels. It side-stepped the national health service structures in these countries as they were failing the people he wanted to help. They were dysfunctional and Joost wanted to start something fresh. This would perform in a very distinct manner and not have the baggage that the national health systems carried with them.

Healthy Entrepreneurs is headquartered in Utrecht, in central Netherlands. The headquarters facilitate the operations of the offices in Congo, Uganda, Tanzania, Ghana and Haiti. They also are building a sophisticated supply chain of reliable and affordable health impact products to serve variety of customers: franchise entrepreneurs, wholesale customers like hospitals, NGOs, and governments.

Joost has invented a new end-to-end supply chain by connecting locally-run and centrally coordinated purchasing structures. These structures sell the highest quality generic medications via independently operated warehouses that are monitored by HE. He has paired this with reliable distribution through local, sustainable micro-health businesses. They believe in regular replenishment of goods and training on Safe Reproductive Health and entrepreneurship and timely provision of promotional materials, bicycle, boxes etc. HE identifies potential entrepreneurs with a secondary school diploma at a minimum, some basic health knowledge and preferably women to setup their own mini-pharmacies.

Joost set up cooperatives to buy medicines and health products straight from suppliers after a thorough quality check. This was vital to bargain on price. But the healthcare is delivered by small entrepreneurial micro-health providers that worked in their local community. The entrepreneur spends $40 in advance and receives a kit containing a solar-powered tablet to educate the local community, order goods and promote new medical products. This mini-pharmacy purchases health goods on credit from HE. The goods are to be paid back within a year of purchase.

This method ensures that the supply chain can be monitored for quality, while the people on the ground, in the community, could give effective advice and care to people that had never received this kind of support before. It is like a franchise system, but where everyone wins. The local franchise holders are just that - local. This means that they get the training and support needed to start their own business that helps their own community. They are also trained on how to educate and consult their community about the products they sell. The effect is that people engage with this more because they are speaking to others that they know and trust. The education forms a large part of the process, so the patients are to look after themselves and remain independent far more effectively. The motivation levels are high because people see each other on a much more regular basis.

The social and financial implications of this model are manifold. For the community, it leads to greater health awareness, behavioral changes and reduction of burden on hospitals. Financially, the system encourages entrepreneurship, creates multiple job opportunities and generates sustainable higher incomes for everyone involved. On the healthcare front, there is reduction of counterfeit products and generation of avenues for new, affordable and reliable products for the end user.

The retention rates for these franchises is as high as ninety-seven percent, so people are seeing this as a viable business opportunity as well as a way to help their own community. People are looked after by Joost van Engen and his team, so they can go out there with the confidence that they are giving the right advice and using medicines that are not counterfeit. Trained entrepreneurs deliver important healthcare advice and accomplish the last-mile delivery.

The future for healthcare is a little cloudy at the moment, but one thing is for sure: the model that is currently being used needs to make an exit. It is not fit for purpose. If new players can be introduced to the market, then the game changes. The pressure is relieved from hospitals to do what they do best. It will take some time for all of this to come through the system, but consider that this initiative of HE has already helped over 3,20,000 people with their sexual education and 1,00,000 have been consulted on contraception. These are lives that are being changed by a sustainable model of business. By 2018, Healthy Entrepreneurs worked with 3650 micro-entrepreneurs and 3000 people per entrepreneur. This resulted in reaching 2.8 million people in five countries since its advent.

Joost's aim now is on partnering with complementary partners and to specialize in developing a wider product range, and building the logistics and technology support. In addition to that, the team is strengthening the franchise network by supporting the financing of flow of goods and sharing all experience/knowledge to support growth. Joost has tied up with companies like Simavi and AidsFonds to create the knowledge base for sexual health education and awareness. Together, they aim to bring about behavioral changes that will reduce diseases like AIDS.

In the future, Healthy Entrepreneurs aims to have four wholesale operations and four thousand entrepreneurs, bringing more innovations to the target market. The goal of Healthy Entrepreneurs is to train entrepreneurs and equip them with innovative and practical solutions that fit the health needs of families in remote areas, while maintaining the right balance between purchasing power and operational expenses.

We need more people like Joost van Engen to think outside the box when it comes to the provision of healthcare. There are so many different solutions out there. We need to be far more collaborative than we presently are and engage with new participants to deliver better healthcare to everyone on the planet. When people of local communities get involved directly, the playground becomes level and grows horizontally. The trust is higher and the rapport is greater bringing the extra edge to sustainability. Unsuspecting new players can make a difference to their own lives, on the health and wealth fronts, while positively impacting the society at large. All of this is possible when people like Joost look at the pyramid bottom-up.

A change in perspective is all that is needed.

SOLUTIONS PRESENT THEMSELVES IN THE MOST UNLIKELY PLACES

The Story of Frank Hofmann and Discovering Hands

Does innovation always mean new technologies or tools? Why cannot innovation also be a new way of looking for things instead, in places where we have never looked before.

Frank Hofmann is an innovator who has looked at a global problem through a very different lens. He has focused on breast cancer and found an extremely powerful, yet simple, way to diagnose breast cancer before it's too late.

Breast cancer is the most frequent cancer in women globally. Nearly two million new cases were diagnosed in 2018 alone. As we are aware, few options for treatment and no exact measures are available to prevent cancer. The more women learn about how to check their breasts and what to look for, the more they are able to bring their concerns to the medical community much earlier and receive a better prognosis. Over the last few decades, there have been public information drives regarding breast cancer in many parts of the world. This has come about because doctors have realized the early detection of the disease brings with it a much higher rate of survival.

The current examination for breast cancer, however, is an expensive one. A mammogram plus an MRI is recommended by the American Cancer Society in women who are at a high risk of being diagnosed with breast cancer starting at the age of thirty. In addition, it doesn't recommend clinical breast examination even in average-risk women for lack of advantage over mammography. Imagine doing these tests each year right from the age of thirty for as long as you live. Not just the cost, the amount of radiation exposure that a woman will accumulate is huge. And this is just for screening. For women between thirty-fifty, where mammography is not recommended, clinical breast examination remains the method of choice.

In parts of the world where the latest detection methods are used, the cost can run into thousands of dollars. And not all healthcare policies pay out to women who have this examination. In Germany, medical insurance covers what is classified as a 'normal' breast examination. Some women end up choosing between their health and their finances; this isn't a great place to be. We use greater detection methods for many diseases, but the cost can deter many families and most medical insurance companies, and hence potential cancer patients are restricted from using them. It is a catch 22 situation that nobody wants to be in.

A study published in the Journal of Women's Health in 2011 concluded that although mammography has been established as a more accurate method of detecting breast cancer, due to the falsely negative reports and missed cancers that still occur, patient-reported breast signs that might indicate a breast cancer must be thoroughly investigated. A self-breast exam remains one of the easiest and most affordable ways to detect a breast cancer early.

Dr. Frank Hofmann looked at the rising cost of breast screening and decided that the future needs to look to help people in a more natural way. Besides making decisions about doing what is best for your body, the cost has to weigh in there somewhere. Patients who choose not to look after their body for reasons of ignorance don't have an easy time. Patients who cannot access healthcare because of cost are also left behind.

Dr. Hofmann pioneered a diagnostically superior, personalized, low-cost breast examination method by training visually impaired people as skilled diagnosticians. The doctor's approach integrates them into the primary health care infrastructure, while enhancing women's healthcare experience and opening an entirely new professional path to a differently-abled constituency.

Discovering Hands was set up with this goal. Dr. Hofmann found that visually impaired women were incredibly able, when trained, at finding cancerous lumps in the breasts of other women. This was the low-cost alternative that he had been looking for. Looking outside of the medical community for an answer may have been daunting at first. He risked ridicule because the detection rates with doctors were very good.

Blind or visually impaired women were trained as Medical Tactile Examiners (MTEs) and got to work with special color-coded patented braille strips to detect lumps in the breast of women with a high degree of accuracy. The cost of these MTEs was far less than the cost of seeing an oncologist. These were examinations that were accurate, personal and were delivered with care and attention. They were overseen by a medically qualified doctor. It has reduced the cost of breast cancer detection by four times from the normal mammography examination i.e., this test can now be availed at only at 30 EUR (US $45) per breast. One such MTE saved the life of Heike Gothe, in her own words.

While still coming to terms with the untimely loss of her husband from illness, Gothe took charge of the family business, a small but successful international export firm in Germany. Not too long after, she received her diagnosis of breast cancer. She had felt a lump in her right breast when she consulted a doctor who confirmed a 12mm lump of cancer. The ultrasound and the mammograms didn't detect another much smaller lump of cancer, just the MTE. The size was 2mm. Gothe says she can sleep in peace thanks to the half-yearly medical examinations she does with the MTEs and can focus her energy on the business. 'I am in good hands,' she says. Quite literally.

Another great advantage of this model is transforming disability into capability. This model uses visually impaired women who otherwise find it difficult to get employed. Their superior sensitive touch along with MTEs training, these women gave a higher precision rate than an average doctor. As to support this clause, a study conducted by Essen University's women's clinic concluded that in '450 cases, MTEs found more and smaller tumors than doctors'. An initial study found that the MTEs were able to detect 28% more and nearly 50% smaller changes in the breasts as comparted to doctors. In fact, tumors just 6-8mm in size, that are more likely to be missed by the average gynecologist doing a breast exam, are twice as likely to be detected by the MTEs.

This thirty-minute breast examination, as compared to the usual three-minute exam, gives women more time to ask questions and be reassured that they are healthy. This involves not only examining the breast, but also educating patients on how to cope with the risk of breast cancer. Discovering Hands is a one-of-its kind organization that is safely, effectively and cost-effectively improving healthcare of women while eliminating the fear attached with breast cancer. Using everyday clinical experiences, the team is not just creating value for the visually impaired, but helping reduce the burden of healthcare on the society in tandem.

The training of MTEs takes place at the BBS Nuremburg, a vocational training center located in South Germany for individuals no longer able to continue their profession as a result of visual impairment or blindness, and at the Discovering Hands owned DH Academy in Berlin. As 'Medical

Tactile Examiners', they participate in a nine-month training program in disability centers, where they learn how to use standardized diagnostic methods for examining female breasts, as well as psychology, communications and administrative skills in medical institutions across Germany. They are examined by a board led by medical doctors and following the examination regulations set up by the North Rhine Medical Association, before they enter the society as breast examiners.

Medical Tactile Examiners are either directly employed by resident doctors or hospitals, or work for different practices and/or hospitals on a freelance basis. The examination is either paid through health insurance [to date, Discovering Hands has agreements with 26 companies in Germany, covering more than 10.3 million women (who can get the examination once a year for free)] or by the patient. They are trained to answer questions that might be weighing on the minds of women undergoing the exam. In fact, these MTEs even teach you how to conduct self-breast exam at home and provide a manual for the same, after finishing their examination.

Dr. Frank Hofmann designed a standardized system of orientation for breast examiners based on braille strips. This mapping system is an innovative solution and has already been adopted by many gynecologists. It consists of five adhesive strips placed around a woman's breast with both braille and color coordinates that allow any abnormality/lump to be pinpointed by two dimensional coordinates. This allows visually impaired women to carry out breast examinations with complete autonomy. Trained as MTEs, a completely new profession that Hofmann created through his standardized training curriculum, they are also able to accomplish other daily tasks of a seeing medical assistant, including the maintenance of medical records.

Post its success in Germany the model was rolled out in other countries as well. Austria has signed the Discovering Hands social franchise contract and pilot projects have been set up in Colombia, Mexico and India. The Netherlands, France, Denmark, Switzerland, UK and Spain have all expressed an interest in the system as well. Dr. Hofmann could be at the forefront of change in the screening of breast cancer for women who may have a decision to make with cost in their mind. The health of the world is far too important to leave in the hands of those who hold the purse strings.

Throughout this book you have read about people that are challenging the way things are done. I suppose that is human nature. We are always inquisitive and always looking for better ways to do things. So many areas of modern life are not constructed in the way we would want or expect if we could build it afresh today. Healthcare is a major area that needs to be reconfigured rather than adapted. We have two routes. One looks to a future of greater healthcare spending in what I deem the wrong places.

Till the year 2018, 42 women who are visually impaired were part of the Discovering Hands network, working in seventeen gynecologists' practices and hospitals across Germany. Within one third of the time invested so far, this number will double. If the goal succeeds in obtaining state recognition for the training program, school leavers can also make the transition to MTE as a primary vocational training course. This will multiply the number of MTEs in Germany in a very short time. More than 1,00,000 examinations have been carried out to date. There are 71,000 cases of breast cancer annually in Germany. Imagine the impact.

For the visually impaired MTEs, this has instilled in them new confidence and have found a place for themselves in society. From being the dependent and slow ones, these MTEs are now independent and not just that, they are actually helping doctors make diagnoses, those with normal vision. The fact that they are actually helping bring peace to other women brings immense joy to them.

Future Plans

* Discovering Hands plans to train approximately 40 more MTEs nationally until 2021, who will have the capacity to carry out a minimum of 38,400 examinations per year.

* In India, Mexico and Colombia, Discovering Hands have pilot projects running with scale-up in planning and are interested in further country roll-out, which operate through a social franchise.

 * It aims to reach 2 million annual examinations all over the world by 2024.

Using tactile diagnostics, the team hopes to be able to detect glaucoma or conduct thyroid exams and detect prostate cancer and testicular cancers in men too someday.

The future for healthcare can be bright if the right steps are taken now. If we keep doing the same things, then we can expect the same results, that is for certain. We are heading along a path that will lead to more of the same. There is no way to adjust the end result if we wait until people are near the end of their timeline before we intervene. By this, I mean that we have to get to meet people before they begin to suffer from an incurable disease, before they have developed complications, before they have something that cannot be reversed. And a solution like Discovering Hands, which on one hand, helps early detection but on the other, creates a respectful job for a person with visual disability is an elegant answer.

Discovering Hands has invited new players into the game. Who would have thought that the visually impaired could detect tumors better than a mammogram or an experienced doctor even? Dr. Hofmann changed the perspective to the problem: instead of focusing on treatment of breast cancer, he looked at how the diagnostics could be improved. This novel approach shows that reflecting at every aspect of a problem is extremely important. Answers might be available at unthought of avenues if only one is willing to give it a thought and honest shot.

CHANGING THE RULES OF THE GAME

Old rules will lead to same solutions, change them

CHANGING THE RULES OF THE GAME

Every healthcare player is in the business of changing mindsets and behavior. The sooner we realize this, the faster we will move toward our end goal. Today our focus is on better diagnosis, faster and cheaper cure and the desire for the Holy Grail to solve all our problems. But what we seem to be missing is that we are already late if we treat health problems after they set in.

The ultimate aim is to make the diseases preventable, and to change behaviors that would curb the diseases from their very roots. The public health campaigns of the past revolving around safe drinking water, immunization and safe sex have contributed to far more significant changes in our lives than better medicines, better hospitals or better diagnostics.

However, healthcare has been stuck in the same old mindset for centuries of detecting a disease early and providing the best medicines to ensure a speedy recovery. There is some shift in the recent years to prevention, but the focus is still on early diagnosis rather than true prevention. This has led to an inordinate number of people getting health checks done on regular basis in the hope of detecting things earlier. While the focus should have been on 'what are the behavioral changes needed now to prevent issues in the future?'

Is this really possible? A world where each person takes optimal possible care of himself and his family to prevent diseases and a disease is as rare as it once used to be. There was a time when cancers were so rare, they used to breed fear in the heart of the people by their mere mention. Cut to today, every family has a member or close friend that has cancer.

In this section you will read about Gamechangers redefining the rules of the game and helping change mindsets.

Nalini and her organization Arogya is helping build a culture of wellbeing via corporate challenges and public recognition. You will also learn about how Dr. Vera Cordeiro and her colleagues are addressing the root causes of ill health via multi-pronged approach of poverty, rights and living conditions. And lastly, about how Dr. Mark Swift and his team are integrating social prescriptions including ballroom dancing and standard of care in medical practices in the UK.

Nalini Saligram realized that peer pressure is a greater force than any authority or pep talk. Using health challenges for employees and their companies to compete in and complete, she is changing the way people look at corporate wellness. Since office is where we spend most of our time today, it is important that health is taken seriously here. Strong steps taken by employers towards better employee health are rewarded in a unique award show held by Arogya each year. This motivates other firms to take that extra step towards being an Arogya-recognized workplace. Healthy employees are good for business after all. Win-win for everyone, don't you think?

Dr. Vera Cordeiro, through her institution Saude Crianca, is changing the way doctors treat patients; she and her team don't just help the patients navigate in the health system, but actually peep into their homes and provide other things that are obstructing good health. Knowing that poverty is a leading cause of disease and death, especially in children, Dr. Vera is fighting to change the entire milieu in which children and their families are raised such that they can be raised healthier, and actually survive childhood. One of the most challenging times in a person's life, one must get through childhood hale and hearty if one must live to be an adult who not just enjoys life, but contributes to the society too. Saude Crianca is aiming to bring change in this very tender age, firmly set in healthy behaviors and educate to prevent disease, not only taking care of the child but also supporting the whole family regarding health, education, income generation, housing and citizenship.

Human beings are social animals, there is no denying this fact. Dr. Swift saw the impact of social activities in today's lives, rather their lack of. He found that social activities can immensely prevent and treat diseases, especially in the mental health domain. In an increasingly aging population, mental health cannot be ignored. His social prescriptions of activities ranging from dancing to hiking to learning a new skill is changing the lives of many people and not just mentally, physically too.

What shifts when we change the rules of the game?

Framework: Increasing patient knowledge and incorporating interventions to target behavioral change

When we start looking outside the frame of the four walls of a hospital, our perspective broadens and we can see newer avenues of bringing in change. Targeting the behavior of persons such that they can themselves eliminate the need to enter into the frame of treatment is truly a paradigm shift that needs to be achieved. Steps towards building the right attitude towards health need to be taken much earlier before disease sets in. When the attitude towards health changes and the person himself is involved with or without the healthcare provider, that's when prevention truly begins.

Policy: Establishing rules and regulations to create a physical or social environment of change

New rules mean new outcomes. When rules are established towards an outcome of health maintenance and prevention of disease, automatically behaviors change to manifest this. When policies reflect political will towards individual health rather than focusing on the economics of health, visibly the focus shifts inside: inside the home, inside the community, inside the relationships, outside the hospital.

CONNECTING WITH EDUCATORS AND WORKPLACES

The Story of Nalini Saligram and Arogya World

Healthcare has been developing along a single line for centuries. We look to help people far too late in the process to have any meaningful intervention. Once someone presents with type 2 diabetes, for example, then the horse has already bolted. Not only are all attempts from then on about managing a disease rather than curing it, but the time and money needed to do this by far outweighs earlier intervention. It would test the skill of any doctor to not only perform an operation or prescribe the right treatment, but also motivate people to do the right things. This is actually one of the key elements in changing behaviors. I believe that there are two strands to this:

* The education to understand what affects health and how to act.
* The motivation to put this education into action.

Telling is speaking to the brain. It is pointing someone in the right direction. It is cold and hard. Selling is speaking to the heart. It gets people off their seat and interested in what you have to say.

Medicine is almost completely focused on the telling part. We tell people to stop smoking. We tell people to lose weight. We tell people to get more exercise. We tell people to cut down on alcohol, sugar, salt and many other things. But we don't sell often enough. Once again, we see an area of healthcare that doesn't perform in an optimal way. People may understand all the 'tell' arguments you give them, but without the 'sell' motivation to do anything, you are wasting your breath. Behavioral change comes when something hits home, i.e., the heart. Research has found that it is easier to quit smoking cold turkey when setting afoot on a religious pilgrimage than it is all life. Why? The answer lies in the heart. Religion is followed by the heart, not by the brain.

We have also seen how moving care away from the daunting and centralized hospital into the community has a big impact on the consumption of healthcare. So why do we insist on excluding people from the conversation?

Communication is vital to reach people earlier in the cycle of wellness. But without the right techniques to reach people, these attempts will not be as effective as they can be. Just communicating with people in their own environment is a step in the right direction, but it needs to be effective to make the kind of sea change that is required.

Take Nalini Saligram's work in India.

Diabetes is a problem across India, with a population of over a billion people and a large majority of those having little access to healthcare education. Add into the mix the poverty that is rife in many parts of the country and you have a problem that is bubbling up for the near future. And it isn't just the poorer people that are facing issues. The growing middle class in the country are working longer hours and consuming an ever-poorer diet. Conditions like type 2 diabetes and heart disease are affecting the people of India in bigger numbers each year.

An estimated 20% of Indians have at least one chronic condition. Sixty-nine plus million Indians live with diabetes, seventy million are said to have pre-diabetes and the number of diabetics is expected to surpass one hundred million by the year 2030. One million die from diabetes each year in India.

Fortunately, diabetes is preventable. According to the World Health Organization (WHO), 80% of diabetes, 80% heart disease and 40% cancers are preventable with three lifestyle changes: avoiding tobacco, eating right, and increasing physical activity. Now, Nalini Saligram could have looked at this as a tell situation. She could have used her background to tell people all the right things that they should be doing. She could have told women that their families' habits had to change. But this would have fallen on deaf ears because people are resistant to being told what to do. Behavior change is the holy grail of diabetes prevention; it is very difficult to do.

So, she looked for a different approach.

She looked at a multi-pronged community approach, taking prevention to where people live and learn and work.

Arogya World's Healthy Schools program targets adolescents, aged eleven to fourteen. The comprehensive two-year program includes classroom and school-based activities, as well as outreach in students' homes and communities. Each year compelling age-appropriate games and learning activities are implemented by trained student leaders or peers. The program's effectiveness is measured through pre- and post-intervention comparisons of the students' self-reported knowledge, attitudes and behaviors. The knowledge about diabetes, its risk factors and healthy behaviors to treat it; physical activity and healthy eating all increased significantly at the end of the study as did the knowledge that diabetes is preventable.

Data reported during the first year of a pilot program conducted in schools in Delhi, India between May 2011 and March 2012 (n=2,263) showed an increase in the daily intake of vegetables from 61.2% to 76.9%. 77.2% students understood that unhealthy eating habits can put you at risk for diabetes as compared to 65.4% at baseline. 61.3% of students reported that being physically inactive can put one at risk for diabetes as compared to 50.1% at the start of the study. Overall impact on improved health behaviors from the pilot program was estimated to be fourteen percent. Nalini and the Arogya team are now scaling up this program to reach hundreds of thousands of urban and rural school children in partnership with many organizations including Hans Foundation, Agastya International Foundation and Ashoka's Nourishing Schools program.

The easiest place to connect with people who are open to ideas and forming their opinions about the world is in schools. Reaching children before their lifestyle habits are set, Nalini believes is smart. But for those that had already passed though the school system, Nalini had to find a different approach. Dragging people back to the classroom was never going to work. Instead she met the women at their homes and others at their workplace.

Through their commitment to the United Nation's Every Woman, Every Child Initiative, Arogya World is committed to improving the health of children as well as women everywhere. They committed (2014) and have fulfilled (2019) their target of teaching additional 10,000 children their two-year Diabetes Prevention Program.

Arogya World targets workplaces for chronic disease prevention because work is where so many people spend a large part of their day. India is a young country with 2/3rds of its population under the age of thirty-five and the 'population pyramid is expected to bulge across the 15-64 age bracket over the next decade, increasing the working age population from approximately 761 million to 869 million during 2011-2020'. [FICCI, EY, 2014]. Many of these employees have sedentary jobs with long, unpredictable hours compounded by long commutes and stress. Arogya World is building an ecosystem of companies in India interested in employee health and wellness.

However, the twist is in the way this is accomplished.

Positive news, recognition and encouragement are prime drivers of behavior change, as important as avoidance of pain and suffering. Nalini understands this very well and is pushing the envelope with her 'Healthy Workplaces Awards'.

Each year in advance of World Diabetes Day, held on 14 November every year, Arogya World holds an annual conference and award event that discusses key issues in workplace health followed by an award ceremony that recognizes organizations for their championship of workplace health. Now in its fifth year, this program and awards attracts the best and biggest employers in India to apply, benchmark themselves and follow through on their commitments to make their environments and their employees' lifestyle healthier.

In 2018, Arogya World recognized and awarded fifteen such companies in India that have put employee health at the forefront in every manner. Stellar speakers from various fields like sleep, lifestyle and mental health were invited to speak about the impact on these at the workplace and how to better them. The awards act as incentives for the organizations to take a more data-driven approach to the health of their employees. This also pushes the employees to take a closer look at their health and take better control.

The robust criteria that mark a company as healthy were co-created with industry in 2012 to ensure they are viable in the real world: http://arogyaworld.org/healthy-workplaces-criteria/. And these are used by Arogya World in a direct and transparent in-person assessment process to select the Healthy Workplaces; some one hundred organizations, large and small, spanning more than two million employees in multiple industries in the public and private sectors. More than twenty-two companies, from multiple sectors are now a part of Healthy Workplaces. Doing so, it has reached 2.3 million employees.

Nalini knows how to go to the heart of the matter. Arogya World has designed programs that go to where all nutritional habits of a home originate: the women. By communicating directly with the women, she is changing their as well their entire household's nutritional habits. In particular, they are changing the way the mother delivers nutrition and teaches her children about healthy food and lifestyle habits. This is directly changing the way the next generation will behave and more likely to have healthier habits right from childhood.

Another step in this journey of raising healthier generations, is teaching the adolescents, children between eleven and thirteen, an age where habits for adulthood are forming. By catching them young, there is a high chance that these adolescents will carry these healthy habits into adulthood, well before they form the bad ones. She designed educational games and activities to package boring health-related information into fun for the children, the very children who are the future workforce of the country.

But what about those who have already been diagnosed with a disease? To address this issue an innovative program that Arogya World deployed was the mDiabetes program where text messages were delivered to over 1 million people in 2012 in collaboration with Nokia Life. mDiabetes went on to become the largest diabetes prevention mobile health program ever done in the world. In collaboration with Emory University they developed the content of these messages to bring about the intended behavioral changes. Ipsos helped test the impact of these messages in simulation and real-world scenarios. For six months, twice a week, messages were sent to persons that enrolled in the program from across India. 56 messages were sent in 12 languages to the participants, in their language of choice.

A detailed analysis of 611 people from the intervention group and 632 from the control group enrolled for the program found that there were statistically significant changes that the text messages brought about at the end of the program. An 11% increase in exercise, 8% increase in consumption of vegetables and 15% hike in consumption of fruits occurred in the participants who received the messages as compared to the control group. 20.95% participants in the intervention group as compared to only 11.55% participants in the control group increased 2 or more healthy behaviors at the end of the 6-month program. Over 150,000 people were helped to lead a healthier life through mDiabetes. These are important steps towards diabetes prevention that improved blood sugar control in participants significantly. Currently, Arogya World is working on mHealth 2.0 and building addition content on complications of diabetes and ways to prevent them, incorporating information about heart disease, cholesterol, kidney disease, and dietary habits to address these concerns.

Nalini Saligram thought about the message she wanted to deliver. It had to be engaging and work in a way different to what had gone before. People across the world brush against healthcare advice but don't pick it up. They sort of understand a little of what is required but don't pull it together in the form of lifestyle changes. Nalini and Arogya World spoke to people in a 'sell' way that made them understand the importance of eating right, but also motivated people to actually go out there and do it.

Nalini changed the rules of the game. Why repeat what most of us have already heard from a friend, relative, newspaper or blog? She showed that simply changing the way the information was being shared to a person changed their reaction to it. Instead of becoming yet another healthcare teacher, she became an ally of the patient in the better health game. Not just in India, Arogya World is also developing programs for Indians in USA to move towards better control over diabetes and other non-communicable diseases like heart disease.

The world of healthcare needs to follow this model. It has many of the elements that we look at in this series on Healthcare Gamechangers:

* It empowers people to take responsibility of their own health

* It takes healthcare out of the four walls of the hospital and into the community

* It connects with educators and employers to deliver effective healthcare

* It shifts attitudes from illness to wellness and on to healthy living

Essentially, it changes nearly every rule of the game as we know it today. Sometimes, it is important to not just look at the start or the end of the communication chain, but also at the fine line that connects these two ends. The way Arogya World has done.

Nalini knows where she is headed and has shown proof of concept. To scale up she is looking to make her programs sustainable, work with large partners and expand her community-based approach to prevention in other geographies. We hope she is successful as India's next generation needs similar programs to stay healthy.

PRIMARY HEALTHCARE IS CARE FIRST, HEALTH SECOND

The Story of Dr. Vera Cordeiro and Saude Crianca

'Healthcare is a broader concept than what traditional medicine advocates.
I believe, in the future, besides the patients' physical health, the living conditions in which they are inserted will be very important, as important as the actual medical diagnosis and treatment'

Dr. Vera Cordeiro

When you tell people how to look after their health, you gain certain results. Using tried and trusted techniques to deal with health issues or illnesses is one way to help people get better. If a patient presents with a certain illness, usually the medical practitioner will often give the same solution to each and every patient that turns up with that issue. It often isn't until the same patient presents with the same issue time and again that the physician looks at the situation in a different light. They then start to look at the root cause of the problem and see if they can deliver any insight on how to change that. At the same time, many doctors don't have links to other professionals, the means to deliver a holistic solution or the time to investigate further. This means that the patient is 'patched up' and sent back out into the world again.

Not only is this approach something that isn't right for the patient, it is actually a far less cost-effective way of delivering healthcare to people. A person coming back time and again to receive the same prescription or advice for the same healthcare problem, doesn't do them or their life justice. It is merely dealing with the symptoms rather than investigating the root cause. This is even more futile when you see members of the same family repeatedly going back to a medical practice for problems that can be linked to the same root cause.

In the modern day of doctor-patient confidentiality and the computerization of medical records, there is little chance of a whole family visiting a practice for advice, or the merry-go-round of doctors being able to spot and act upon a root cause from people who live in the same place. The 'sticking plaster' solution gets people back on their feet again and allows them to get on with their life until the next illness crops up, but does nothing to provide or promote an environment that makes these illnesses less likely. In many parts of the world, especially the poorer parts, there has to be a sea change in how medicine is administered. This is where pioneers like Vera Cordeiro come in.

Saúde Criança Association (ASC), is an independent social organization founded by Dr. Vera Cordeiro in 1991 in Rio de Janeiro, Brazil that pioneered an innovative methodology to assist poor families that have a sick child undergoing treatment at a public health facility. The crisis becomes real when the pre-existing challenges of poverty worsen with the need to care for the child's health, threatening the family's integrity even further. ASC promotes self-sufficiency of Brazilian families with children suffering from acute and chronic disease typically linked with poverty.

Saúde Criança's program, the 'Family Action Plan' (FAP), adopts an innovative methodology: it is based on the principle that poverty is one of the important causes of disease. The causes of poverty and illness are multidimensional. The plan, which consists of a multidisciplinary team exerts integrated actions in the areas of health, education, citizenship, housing, and income, and is built based on each family's needs. Besides overcoming the immediate difficulties inherent to the child's post-hospitalization phase, the entity's goal is to offer orientation and opportunities so that the family unit has its rights guaranteed and can enjoy a reasonable quality of life.

Saúde Criança fights for social inclusion by promoting human development.

The crucial element of the methodology and one of the keys to its success is the family's active participation elaborating the plan, objectives, and goals to be met during each phase over the two years in which it is part of the program. Every family is assisted individually, according to their needs and potential, during a period of approximately two years. The family's progress is tracked during regular meetings with the Saúde Criança team with the objective of helping the family achieve dignity and autonomy.

In alignment with the World Health Organization's definition of health, Dr. Vera feels that, 'Healthcare is the promotion, prevention and maintenance of health as well as the diagnosis and treatment of diseases that can affect the human being.

'In this field of knowledge, it is very important to promote biopsychosocial well-being. And for this to happen, it is not only necessary that the patient is extensively analyzed as per traditional medical knowledge, but also through a lens that allows various levels of diagnosis and treatment including spiritual and psychological development, and knowledge of the conditions of life to which the patient and their families are submitted.

'Therefore, housing, income generation, education and citizenship are some of the crucial areas that should be integral to the patient's treatment and diagnosis.'

And it is the words 'dignity' and 'autonomy' from the description of what Saude Crianca stand for, from earlier in the chapter, that ring out the loudest when you read on. Being well used to be something that was handed down from one generation to another with the health of the family being considered highly important by the elders as those, that followed would be looking after them in their old age. We now expect specialists to do this for us. The pressures on the budgets of modern medicinal practices mean that the simpler ailments to treat should be a matter of public knowledge, rather than kept a deep and dark secret by the medical community or leaving people to take a chance on the internet and hope the advice they read works.

Dr. Vera Cordeiro founded Saude Crianca in Brazil way back in 1991, which is an age ago in medical terms. Looking back that far, people were dying of cancer where they now survive, heart disease was ravaging the modernized world and we knew only a fraction of what we now know today in just about every area of medicinal science. Saude Crianca was set up with the aim of providing support for families in the poorest parts of Brazil and abroad.

Dr. Cordeiro looked at the medical support for children in particular as being compassionate and effective at the point of contact, but not having the foresight to deal with the issues that brought the children to the attention of the medical community in the first place. The five areas of care that Cordeiro looked at were vital to providing an environment that reduced the chances of becoming ill to begin with:

- Health
- Housing
- Citizenship
- Income

- Education

With all of these areas performing badly, the patient was very likely to be back again soon. The lifestyle of poverty means that people end up in a cycle of illness that is hard to break with pure medicine alone. When all of these areas are taken care of, then the chance of illness becomes much lesser. When you look at it in these terms, it is a clear picture. But in a poor part of Brazil, the doctors have a great deal of pressure on their time. The solution takes time.

Dr. Vera Cordeiro worked for nearly 20 years as a doctor in one of the largest public hospitals in Rio de Janeiro and she was upset and annoyed that much of her hard work was going to waste. She would attend to young children and get them out of a critical situation. Many would present to the hospital she worked in with infectious diseases and through her arduous work and the team around her, she would be in a position to send them home with the disease in check.

But then often, far too often for this modern world, she would see them return with the same disease or find out that they had died from that disease at home. She couldn't keep working along the same lines of fix and fail. She could no longer stand back and watch a system that didn't provide long-lasting results for people. She knew a change had to come. In fact, she knew that she would have to enact this change from outside the current system to stand any chance of making a difference in the life of the kids she treated.

So, with a sense of adventure and the never-say-die spirit she still has today, Dr. Cordeiro sold many of her belongings and set up the not-for-profit organization that is Saude Crianca today. She recruited volunteers and trained them to work with families that needed the extra help and support that would take them away from the cycle of illness-treatment-illness that was widely prevalent. They provided basic supplies that were not present before and built people up enabling them to gain a better control of their own medical destiny. They also sent the families for vocational training courses in order to promote self-sustainability. This is a hands-up that gives people a sense of purpose about their lives, the knowledge that they can manage their family in these five key areas to achieve better results and that word 'autonomy'.

But there were naysayers all along the way who said this would never work. Dr. Cordeiro recalls, 'I remember a few years ago being invited to give a lecture in Switzerland where I showed a poster with the five areas in which we work to show our mission and vision concerning health promotion: health, education, housing, citizenship and income. Listening to the explanation and looking at the poster, a manager from a Swiss bank told me: "I would never invest in your project. This work has no focus." Luckily for me, Muhammad Yunus, a Nobel Peace prize winner, was by my side and told me: 'No matter what you've heard, I tell you, Saúde Criança is a powerful methodology of inclusion for the poorest. You are empowering the head of the family. He does not understand that to strengthen an entire family, and to promote health, action is needed in all these areas.'

Putting families in control of what they do, where they live, what they eat and other factors based on education means they know what they want for themselves and feel confident to go out and get it. The feeling of helplessness is all-consuming in the world that Dr. Cordeiro knew before the program she built was rolled out to the masses. Families just lurched from one disaster to another with the support of the medical community to bandage them and send them back to their prevalent circumstances. No more.

As many diseases are caused by poverty, and poverty is a multidimensional issue, the multidisciplinary work of Saúde Criança is at the heart of social inclusion and the promotion of human development.

The Impact

An Evaluation of Long-Term Impact, conducted by Georgetown University in 2013, analyzed the assisted families three and five years after the Family Action Plan conclusion date. The study revealed a 92% increase in family income, a growth in the number of families that own their own home (before only 26% were owners; after, 50% of the families already owned their own home after the assistance ended), among other indicators.

There was also an 86% reduction in re-entry into the hospital among the evaluated group, with a significant drop in costs for the public health system.

The average hospital stays for children went from 62 days to just under 9 days.

The family's perception of its well-being increased from 9.6%, considered 'Good'/'Very Good', to 51.2%.

The school enrollment of children that enrolled with Saude Crianca shot from a meagre 10% to nearly 92% after the program. In tandem, adult employment went up to 70% from 54%, as healthier kids meant parents could focus more on earning a better livelihood instead of staying home to care for the sick child.

These numbers alone indicate that the Saude Crianca program makes a long-term impact and massive difference to the lives of families it touches and how they interact with the world. Just imagine the pressure this has taken off the doctors of Rio de Janeiro when they turn up for work and have people to deal with that, they know they can help and sustain a longer-term level of health. They have a better knowledge of what Saude Crianca can do for people and feel like they won't see the same person again because of their environment.

The program is building all the time and has become public policy in Belo Horizonte, the sixth largest city in Brazil. It has helped more than 75,000 people directly with the organization starting to look at different markets.

In the words of Dr. Cordeiro: 'During my academic training as a doctor, I did not imagine that in the future, to prevent illness and improve the physical health of children, I would have to hire engineers and architects to improve housing condition of these children and their families, as well as hiring lawyers to support families with sick children struggling for their rights.

'A nurse seeing me working at the hospital and at the same time collecting resources to improve the lives of socially vulnerable families who would be discharged from the hospital asked me: "Besides being a doctor, are you a nun?

What's your real job?" Our institution methodology has been replicated to twenty-three public hospitals in Brazil. Many entrepreneurs who learnt about our work took our DNA to be implemented in Africa, Asia and Europe.'

The future of healthcare for the poorest people must look very differently to how it is being administered in many parts of the world. Firefighting can only do so much. If the conditions that people live in do not change, then results won't change either. Making people aware of the basic issues that affect their health and giving them power over them will make a bigger long-term change to the health of the planet than only prescribing more drugs. It is pioneers like Dr. Cordeiro that will lead the way.

The idea behind much of what Dr. Cordeiro does is one that has a fundamental connection to the saying:

'Give a man a fish and he will eat for a day. Teach him how to fish and he will eat forever'.

It is a principle that permeates many aspects of one's life. We are given so much by so many people, that the notion of learning how to do something yourself doesn't feel natural in some areas. Healthcare is one of these. People who practice alternative medicine or websites that show people how to 'cure' ailments themselves are labelled as dangerous to the health of many. The internet is far too full of information and it is almost impossible to separate the good from the bad. If you say something with a convincing enough tone then people will interpret it as the gospel truth. But healthcare professionals of the past twenty years or so are as guilty as the website doctors. They haven't given people sound advice on how to manage their health. They have just given the magic bullet and moved on to the next in line. The mindset of patients being customers and people waiting to be helped as people waiting to be seen has to alter. Thus, the modern mantra should be: 'Give a man a prescription and he will be well for a while. Teach him how to manage his health and he will be well for life'.

'Our goal for the next ten years is for our methodology to become public policy throughout Brazil. Another way to scale is through a coalition of national and international institutions that will implement the family action plan (FAP) not only in our country but also abroad.,' says Dr. Cordeiro.

REIMAGINING PRESCRIPTIONS

The Story of Mark Swift and Social Prescribing

P lacing people at the heart of healthcare has lost its way over the last twenty years or so. In fact, only recently have we started to talk about patient centric care. As healthcare services became more accessible to larger populations, the obvious solution, at the time, was viewed as moving healthcare provisions along the same lines as many other industries. Service business has changed with the advent of mass production and mass communication. Other businesses have been able to serve more people in shorter time with lower costs. The rise of the internet and social media has made this effect even more marked.

But while the number of people being served has gone up exponentially, the service levels received have dropped through the floor. Other businesses like banking and telecom had to innovate rapidly to handle this paradox: serving more people while maintaining better quality. They invested in automation, ERP systems, strict protocols for managing customer processes and decentralized decision making. Adopting the same model of serving more people in a short time in the healthcare sector has also led to declining standards of care that have not been consistent with what people might have expected not too long ago. The profit levels of healthcare and pharmaceutical companies have driven up, but the customers are inevitably the ones that have suffered as a result of all this drive for greater profit margins and higher numbers of 'patients seen'.

As we have looked at in previous chapters, the fact that more people are seen for a shorter period of time in the short-term only presents long-term issues that will swamp the healthcare provider market. The population is getting older and, quite frankly, as levels of poverty and inequality rise they create divides between those with good health and those without. Across the globe, the future map for healthcare provision is being planned. The solutions seem to be of greater resources, greater expenses and a more efficient way of pushing these numbers through. This makes the problem one that will get bigger all the time, rather than it being one that is being tackled effectively.

Doing the same thing time and time again has proven to be the wrong way to work. If we have a system that doesn't produce the right results for people, then why would we continue doing the same things repeatedly? In business, they define this as insanity. But in medicine we keep at it. We keep giving people a prescription for statins when their readings show a certain level rather than getting people out walking or taking another form of exercise. We experiment with different treatments for Alzheimer's when getting people to learn a new instrument or a new language is seen as a better way to protect and repair those neural pathways that will hold off the disease for longer. The notion of addressing the root cause of why people fall ill in the first place, the social issues that lead to illness like debt, stigma, loneliness and poverty, and act as barriers to health need to be addressed too.

Based in the northwest of England, Mark Swift looked at how the care of people in his community was delivered. Working with colleagues in the NHS, and with local citizens he analyzed the healthcare profile of his local community in Halton and considered the fact that they had an aging population, significant levels of poverty and deprivation and that people were increasingly reliant on the medical community for their health and wellbeing. People presented to their GP with ailments that were caused or exacerbated by their social circumstances for which lifestyle advice is provided. Many of these ailments could have been easily prevented or treated right at home with the correct social support, education and medical advice.

The power was completely in the hands of the medical teams who would diagnose, hand out prescriptions and send people off for treatment in their role as all-powerful authority on all-things healthcare. But they were not as powerful when it came to making decisions. Healthcare professionals are disincentivized from, and ill-equipped to, scrape beyond the surface of a health problem. They may have been trained to look at the whole patient at med school, but out in the real world, doctors and nurses followed a set of guidelines that states how to act in certain situations. And the solutions were pretty much all chemical. Alongside regular advice to lose weight and stop smoking, GPs handed out prescriptions. People felt better. But in the short term.

Swift identified the patterns that put a lot of pressure on the resources of the local healthcare provisions. Considered one of the best models of social healthcare in the world, the National Health Service or NHS in the United Kingdom is funded by the taxpayer and is free at the point of service. From when it was launched in 1948 with a budget of £437 million to spend, today the NHS as a budget or £124.7 billion (2017-18) to provide medical aid to the society. So, they have to ensure that they are spending taxpayers' money in the most efficient way.

The NHS often ends up being a political football as the aging population, growing levels of deprivation and ever-expanding range of treatments mean that more money is requested for this service every year. And this would put it on the same path as many other health provisions across the world.

Through a program labelled Social Prescribing, the team under Swift looked at how they could develop the education of people in the community so they lead to timely consultations with doctor rather than clogging up the healthcare system with ailments that could have been treated at home, or even worse, end up with a totally preventable disease because they didn't know the effect their lifestyle was having on their body.

The team looked at four main areas:

- What social models of healthcare can be used

- What are the determinants of health, particularly on a local level

- Putting together and delivering interventions that could be shown to work

- Remodeling existing healthcare pathways to take these new interventions into account

So, they look at the determinants that are causing the most strain on their healthcare provision. These can be very different in each part of England and each part of the world. The demographics and environmental factors involved mean that each area is different. Diverse issues need diverse solutions.

Prescribing a medicine seems like a magic bullet for patients, it does two things that make it feel transactional:

- The patient walks away with something physical that they believe will help their symptoms

- The doctor can quickly move on to the next patient, knowing that the person they have just seen is happy

But the solution here is putting out fires rather than giving the education that will stop fires in the future. So, Mark Swift and his team have opened up their practices to prescribing things other than drugs. The models they have developed at Wellbeing Enterprises have been co-designed and developed with doctors, patients and wider stakeholders.

The GPs and associated medical teams are very mindful of the limitations of medicine. Indeed, one GP said of this, 'I often feel like I'm applying a sticking plaster to a much bigger problem.'

Of the models they have codeveloped, clinicians have said, 'The services have become as effective as the prescription pad in reaching out to the social circumstances of people's lives.' Clinicians can now prescribe:

Nordic walking

Tango dancing

Gardening

Life skills courses

Confidence classes

Stress management

Mindfulness

Creative crafts

Sleep and relaxation

Singing and comedy

Emotional awareness

Volunteering

So, the mindset is changed straightaway from one where the patient expects a pill and where the doctor can only prescribe something from a list of pills. This brings the solutions home in a way that advice can only do so much with. If we delegate responsibility for health solely to the individual, then we let governments off the hook in terms of policies that condemn people to live in poverty and consequently, poor health.

Wellbeing Enterprises addresses the root causes of poor health, develops strategies to address these issues, alongside providing health promoting interventions and educational support. Further to that. WE joins forces with other organizations to push for a social movement for more progressive government policies that address grotesque levels of inequality.

Dr. Lynne Freidli, author of the WHO's 'Mental Health, resilience and inequalities report', heartily endorses the social prescribing program and their ongoing commitment to genuine partnership with local communities.

A prescription has become the all-powerful solution in society to a problem. People are not happy until they walk away from the doctor with a piece of paper that is supposed to carry the solution. Many people have stopped going to see their doctor because they are told on every visit to stop smoking and lose weight. This has been turned around where people can get classes and nicotine patches on prescription to help them stop smoking. The results have been very positive. Now if people are prescribed dancing classes to keep them fit and active, they get to walk away with that piece of paper but it doesn't only lead to someone popping a pill.

Doctors can have that conversation about losing weight, but not with one eye on the clock and the thought that their words will have no impact. They can prescribe some Nordic walking along with a life skills training class so their patient will be able to fully understand the benefits of exercise and eating the right things. They can pass their patient over to someone who they know and trust will deliver a solution. The training looks at setting goals, changing attitudes and pledging to get better. These are far more powerful tools in the fight against disease and illness than giving out another prescription for pills. It allows the healthcare team to focus instead on a population that feels better and can do something about changing their own life, rather than being in the hands of the doctor for anything related to how they feel. It is typically a combination of the two; by medicine and 'social' health working together they can augment outcomes, aid recovery and reduce demand on services.

There are various key factors that strengthen the Wellbeing program crafted by Mark Swift and the team. For a holistic health approach, they started by carrying out a needs-assessment of the Halton community and not only identified the population needs, but also patient level needs. They acknowledged the social inequalities, inequities and social determinants of health that shape the face of public health. They involved the Board of Directors of the Halton Clinical Commissioning Group (CCG) and presented their insights on a community-centered model of health. The Wellbeing Enterprises Staff also collaborated with public health consultants, General Practitioners, patients, and the community.

Thus, by involving more stakeholders, they managed to encourage their involvement and interest in healthcare and other cost saving methods. They formed their Key Performance Indicators only after the implementation of the model. This facilitated them to demonstrate the impact of their model with flexibility after trying several approaches to the intervention. The social wellbeing service and the social prescribing service links patients to non-medical sources of support in the community. This service, based on cognitive behavioral approaches, mindfulness, hobby groups and self-care strategies increase patient compliance which could also lead to better medication/pharmacotherapeutic adherence. Thus, it works in complement to the medical interventions and incorporates a physical and mental component to it.

Mark Swift and his team have become very successful at what they do. From Halton, they have spread and now provide services in Knowsley, and St Helens and Liverpool too. They train clinicians and allied professionals in 'social wellbeing approaches' all across the country in order to enhance the quality of clinical provision.

In 2014, they won the NAPC Best Practice 'Health and Wellbeing Innovation of the Year' award. They were one of the first ever non-clinical service to win the award. It is positive testament to the work that they do, and the lives they can benefit. In 2015 they won the prestigious Health Service Journal (HSJ) for this work and its contribution to healthcare innovation.

WE once had a patient who knew to play the ukulele, and so they started running an ukulele class. It took off and the class became so popular that they ran out of ukuleles. Another similar success story is of the tango dancer who started a tango club that helped her and so many others that joined the club. Today, WE holds classes for singing, dancing, guitar, and even knitting. The social impact speaks for itself.

Close to 30,000 people have benefitted from WE as of 2015.

As per their 2016-17 report, WE engaged about 1150 people in 2016-17 alone, 90% persons of which rated the program 8/10 or more. 73% people undertook health promoting activities. 61% and 63% people noted reduction in anxiety and loneliness. 67% people noted an improvement in their overall wellbeing and felt closer to others.

£1,769,987 public spend on healthcare was saved owing to savings in mental health, prescriptions, visits to GPs and physical exercise, and activity.

For every pound invested, a social value of £118.76 was created owing to the social impact the programs created.

Advances in medical procedures, more effective drugs and better work processes have meant that we have kept up with the rising demand for healthcare until the last ten years or so. Now, the pressure is really on to provide the same solutions as today but to many more people in the years to come. The cost of healthcare is rising fast. More treatments mean more reliance on doctors to nurse people back to health that were given a death sentence with a certain diagnosis in the recent past. For instance, around twenty years ago, a massive proportion of patients diagnosed with lung cancer wouldn't survive the year. Now more than half do. This is a great statistic that means more people get to see their children grow up or fulfill more of their dreams. The impact on the life of a person is massive in that respect. But this isn't the long-term road.

The solution where we plough more money into healthcare to keep people alive for longer looks positive from the outside. But it is inevitably unsustainable.

The solution where we teach people how to avoid disease in an engaging way that motivates them to act is a solution that is far more workable for a growing (and aging) population. This solution is being explored by the people I have outlined in this book, and many others in different parts of the world. These social approaches will become ever more important as the divide between rich and poor becomes increasingly larger.

By changing the rules of the prescription game, Mark Swift changed the way patients looked at a prescription and experienced better and different outcomes than ever before.

BIBLIOGRAPHY

Primary care is a team sport:

- http://blogs.umb.edu/gerontologyinstitute/2018/11/28/institute-talk-a-conversation-with-iora-health-ceo-rushika-fernandopulle/

- The Journal of American's Physician Groups. Fall 2018; 12 (3). Available at: https://2h24dy2ehwvl3j7p7q1hih8t-wpengine.netdna-ssl.com/wp-content/uploads/2018/11/JAPG_Colloquium2018_finallores-1.pdf

- https://medium.com/built-by-us/built-by-rushika-fernandopulle-of-iora-health-2e43c5675b30

- https://www.ashoka.org/en-IN/fellow/rushika-fernandopulle

Using the rare point of contact to transform care:

- http://www.noorahealth.org/

- https://www.edexlive.com/people/2018/nov/30/how-noora-health-a-start-up-is-educating-people-to-take-care-of--their-health-and-early-detection-o-4587.html

- https://extreme.stanford.edu/projects/noora-health/

- https://www.changemakers.com/makingmorehealth/entries/noora-health

- https://www.ashoka.org/en-IN/fellow/edith-elliott

End of life care delivered with empathy:

- Kumar S., Numpeli M. Neighborhood network in palliative care. Indian J Palliative Care [serial online] 2005 [cited 2019 Feb 3]; 11:6-9. Available from: http://www.jpalliativecare.com/text.asp?2005/11/1/6/16637

- https://www.worldcancercongress.org/sites/congress/files/slides/Pre0005-Kumar%20Suresh.pdf

Care in your neighborhood:

- https://www.buurtzorg.com/about-us/buurtzorgmodel/

- https://www.ashoka.org/en-IN/fellow/jos-de-blok

Taking the fight to the streets:

- http://carepro.co.jp/wordpress/wp-content/uploads/2015/10/Carepro-FICCI-HEAL.pdf

- https://www.ashoka.org/en-IN/fellow/takashi-kawazoe

Retaining doctors and the faith of the people:

- https://www.changemakers.com/ashoka-fellows/entries/fundaci%C3%B3n-venezolana-para-la-medicina-familiar

- http://www.medicinafamiliar.org/

It takes a community to fix individual health:

- https://www.who.int/news-room/fact-sheets/detail/diabetes

- https://www.idf.org/our-network/regions-members/north-america-and-caribbean/members/66-mexico.html

- https://www.who.int/bulletin/volumes/95/6/17-020617/en/

- https://www.vallartadaily.com/diabetes-in-mexico/

- https://www.ashoka.org/en-IN/fellow/morgan-guerra

Redesigning a business model to reinvent an old one:

- https://www.ashoka.org/en-IN/fellow/joost-van-engen

- https://www.healthyentrepreneurs.nl/

- https://simavi.org/long-read/healthy-business-healthy-lives-from-health-worker-to-entrepreneur/

- https://www.who.int/bulletin/africanhealth/en/

Solutions present themselves in the most unlikely places:

- https://zeroproject.org/practice/discovering-hands-germany/

- https://www.wcrf.org/dietandcancer/cancer-trends/breast-cancer-statistics

- https://www.cancer.org/content/dam/cancer-org/research/cancer-facts-and-statistics/breast-cancer-facts-and-figures/breast-cancer-facts-and-figures-2017-2018.pdf

- Roth MY et al. Self-Detection Remains a Key Method of Breast Cancer Detection for U.S. Women. J Women's Health (Larchmt). 2011 Aug; 20(8): 1135-1139. https://www.ncbi.nlm.nih.gov/pmc/articles/PMC3153870/

- https://www.discovering-hands.de/initiative/hintergruende-ziele/

- https://collectivehub.com/2017/01/how-the-blind-are-changing-cancer-detection-thanks-to-this-social-entrepreneur/

- https://www.bbc.com/news/magazine-31552562

Connecting with educators and workplaces:

- http://arogyaworld.org/

- https://www.ashoka.org/en-IN/fellow/nalini-saligram

- https://www.jmir.org/2016/8/e207/#figure2

Primary healthcare is care first, health second:

- https://www.ashoka.org/en-IN/fellow/vera-regina-gaensly-cordeiro

- http://www.saudecrianca.org.br/en/nosso-trabalho/resultados-de-impacto/

Reimagining prescriptions:

- https://www.kingsfund.org.uk/projects/nhs-in-a-nutshell/nhs-budget

- https://www.nhs.uk/using-the-nhs/about-the-nhs/the-nhs/

- http://www.indiaenvironmentportal.org.in/files/

file/NHP%202018.pdf

- http://www.wellbeingenterprises.org.uk/wp-content/uploads/2015/06/206921-low-res.pdf

- https://www.local.gov.uk/sites/default/files/documents/just-what-doctor-ordered--6c2.pdf

Made in United States
North Haven, CT
13 May 2023